H

SELF-HEALING
FOR WOMEN

THE FAMILY
HOME REMEDIES
COLLECTION

SELF-HEALING
FOR WOMEN

America's top doctors,
therapists and health experts solve
women's unique health problems

**BY THE EDITORS OF
PREVENTION MAGAZINE HEALTH BOOKS**

Rodale Press, Emmaus, Pennsylvania

Copyright © 1995 by Rodale Press, Inc.

Prevention is a registered trademark of Rodale Press, Inc.

Printed in the United States of America on recycled ♻ paper

Book Packager: Sandra J. Taylor
Cover and Book Designer: Eugenie Seidenberg Delaney

Library of Congress Cataloging-in-Publication Data

Self-healing for women : America's top doctors, therapists and health experts
   solve women's unique health problems / by the editors of Prevention Magazine
   Health Books.
      p. cm. — (The Family home remedies collection)
   Includes index.
   ISBN 0–87596–265–3 paperback
      1. Women—Health and hygiene. 2. Self-care, Health.
   I. Prevention Magazine Health Books. II. Series.
   RA778.S475 1995
   613' .04244—dc20   94–24203
                                                          CIP

Distributed in the book trade by St. Martin's Press

2 4 6 8 10 9 7 5 3 1   paperback

Contents

AGE SPOTS

Talk about a spotty reputation! Heck, most people can't agree on what to *call* these unappealing but otherwise harmless dark spots that usually occur on the forehead and the back of the hands and arms.

Some folks think age spots are caused by old age—an understandable mistake, since the spots are extremely common after age 55 and rarely appear before middle age. Others know them as liver spots.

The appearance of these dark, blotchy spots can be scary—resembling the early forms of skin cancer to the untrained eye. But genuine age spots are really nothing more than "adult freckles" that result from overexposure to the sun. (However, if you notice an increase in size or "bizarre" color changes, see your doctor immediately.)

"Age spots should really be called sun spots, because they are caused by being out in the sun," says D'Anne Kleinsmith, M.D., a cosmetic dermatologist at William Beaumont Hospital near Detroit. "They have absolutely nothing to do with your liver and little to do with your age, other than the fact that they usually occur on older people."

Still, they *are* unbecoming. Sometimes they may be raised and look like tiny moles. Usually, though, they're just like dark, smooth freckles. If you've had them, you've probably noticed that they seem to appear suddenly on sun-exposed skin areas (usually areas *not* protected with sunscreen). So here's what to do about liver spots . . . er, age sp . . . uh, *lentigines* (their medical name).

Get help from hydroquinone. This safe "lightening agent" is found in products such as Porcelana and Esoterica that you can obtain without a prescription. Hydroquinone helps lighten age spots until they become unnoticeable. "Dab it on the individual spots with a cotton ball," says Dr. Kleinsmith. This therapy usually takes a month or two before you see any results. Follow the directions on the package and try to dab the medication right on the spots, so you don't "bleach" the pigment in nonaffected skin.

SUNSCREEN EACH DAY KEEPS AGE SPOTS AWAY

The best way to avoid *ever* having age spots is to use a good-quality sunscreen each time you go outdoors, including when it's overcast. And if you already have age spots, sunscreen will keep them from darkening and will help prevent new ones.

Either way, remember the "15" rules.

Look for a sun protection factor (SPF) of at least 15. Unprotected, the average person's skin turns red—a signal of overexposure—after just 30 minutes. But with SPF 15 sunscreen, you can stay out 15 times as long, or seven hours, with the same effect (although it's not recommended).

Apply sunscreen at least 15 minutes before going outdoors. That way, the skin has a chance to absorb it.

Shed away "spotted" skin. Lac-Hydrin Five lotion, a nonprescription remedy, contains lactic acid. "The acid can help bleaching agents work faster by enhancing the normal shedding of upper, 'dead' skin layers," says Michael Ramsey, M.D., a dermatologist and clinical instructor of dermatology at Baylor College of Medicine in Houston. This leaves a lighter layer of skin underneath.

Reach for lemon aid. "The juice of a fresh lemon is acidic enough to safely peel off the upper layer of skin, which will remove or lighten some age spots," says Jerome Z. Litt, M.D., a dermatologist and assistant clinical professor of dermatology at Case Western Reserve University School of Medicine in Cleveland. "Rub it on with a cotton ball twice daily where the age spots are, and in six to eight weeks, they should begin to fade away."

How about an onion rub? Rubbing a piece of sliced red onion on age spots can have the same fading effect, "since it has the same peeling acid as fresh lemon juice," adds Dr. Litt.

Use castor oil for smooth relief. "If the surface of individual lesions appears rougher than surrounding skin—which often occurs with age spots—applying castor oil twice daily with a cotton swab will sometimes bring about improvement," says Dr. Ramsey. On larger lesions, a bandage applied with the castor oil at nighttime may speed improvement.

Be a shady character. "Since age spots are caused by excessive sun exposure, avoid the sun and you'll avoid age spots," says Albert M. Kligman, M.D., Ph.D., a dermatologist and professor of dermatology at the University of Pennsylvania School of Medicine in Philadelphia. "You will never see an age spot on someone who stays in the shade." If you already have age spots, limiting sun exposure will help prevent them from darkening and will minimize a recurrence or the appearance of new ones.

Cover 'em up. If all else fails in trying to remedy them, hide them. "Many types of makeup can cover the spots," says Edward Bondi, M.D., a dermatologist who is affiliated with the University of Pennsylvania Hospital in Philadelphia. "If they are really dark spots, a heavier-based makeup will work, but if they're not so bad, then many water-based types will do the trick. A product called Covermark has routinely been used to hide age spots." *Note*: If you suffer from acne, avoid heavier oil-based makeups, because they can worsen blemishes.

BINGE EATING

T here are generally two triggers to an eating binge: Either you're on a diet and your body needs the extra food or you overeat because you're trying to suppress some emotion—stress, loneliness, depression or anger," says Adam Drewnowski, Ph.D., director of the Human Nutrition Program at the University of Michigan in Ann Arbor. "Either way, the end result is usually feelings of guilt."

While doctors say understanding and resolving your feelings is the best way to get off these feeding frenzies, here's some immediate help.

Write about your feelings. "I tell my patients who binge-eat when they're angry or depressed to write down their feelings in a letter they *don't* intend to send," says Karyn Scher, Ph.D., director of training for the Graduate Hospital Eating Disorders Service in Philadelphia.

"One reason why women are much more likely than men to go on eating binges is because our society has trained them to suppress their anger or other 'negative' emotions. Simply write how you feel, or pen a sample dialogue as you would like it to unfold for two people—yourself and the person causing those feelings," suggests Dr. Scher.

Besides keeping you from bingeing (both your mind and hands are occupied), this technique has another benefit: You'll learn healthier ways to deal with negative emotions.

Antibinge hotline: Call a friend. If you binge-eat out of boredom, it may be a sign of loneliness or social isolation, so Dr. Scher suggests you call a friend or relative. "I tell my patients to create a phone chain with at least six people they can call when they feel lonely or bored."

Count to 20. The next time you get a food craving, make yourself wait 20 minutes before you succumb. Most food cravings that *aren't* due to hunger will subside in that time. If not—if you're still hungry after 20 minutes—then you probably do need food.

"Ideally, you should do something that's incompatible with eating, such as taking a walk," suggests Linda Crawford, a certified eating disorders counselor at Green Mountain at Fox Run, a weight and health management center in Ludlow, Vermont.

Take to the sidewalk. Walking and other forms of aerobic exercise are among the best ways to kill food cravings, adds Dr. Scher. Vigorous exercise may break a cycle of stress-induced bingeing. Lots of people report a sense of physical well-being after 20 minutes of aerobic exercise that offsets the urge to binge.

Drown your sorrows. Even if emotion rather than hunger is driving you to eat, drinking lots of water can help—by freshening your taste buds and filling your belly, which reduces your food cravings, according to George Blackburn, M.D., Ph.D., chief of the Nutrition and Metabolism Laboratory at New England Deaconess Hospital in Boston.

Choose low-fat alternatives. "If you totally deny yourself, you'll go crazy and just binge out even more later on," says Dr. Drewnowski. "Instead of forbidding yourself to eat, indulge in a smaller portion of a lower-fat substitute. For instance, if you're craving a bowl of ice cream, give in to a scoop of frozen yogurt."

Although many people suggest carrying around a bag of carrots or celery sticks for when the munchies hit, Dr. Drewnowski has found that these crunchy substitutes don't work. "You need to eat something along the same lines as what you're craving, only in smaller portions," he advises.

Sizzle your taste buds with spicy foods. Ever try to wolf down mass quantities of chili or peppers, horseradish or curry? It can't be done. So when the urge to eat is overwhelming, reach for a hot Mexican, Thai or Indian snack.

"The flavor is so intense that you'll find yourself eating much smaller portions than you would of bland or sweet foods," says

BE ALERT TO WARNING SIGNS

The signs and symptoms of eating disorders can be subtle and insidious, and can include:

- Distorted body image.
- Excessive exercising.
- Preoccupation with weight and diet.
- Loss of three consecutive menstrual periods.
- Loss of pubic hair.
- Binge eating, especially of "junk" foods.
- Significant weight loss (at least 15 percent below normal).
- Significant weight fluctuations (10 pounds or more a month).
- Inability to recognize basic feelings, such as hunger or sadness.
- Sensitivity to cold.
- Abuse of laxatives, diuretics and emetics.
- Erosion of dental enamel (from gastric acid during vomiting).
- Withdrawal from family and friends.
- Inability to concentrate.
- Depression and loss of sleep.

Maria Simonson, Ph.D., Sc.D., professor emeritus and director of the Health, Weight and Stress Program at the Johns Hopkins Medical Institutions in Baltimore. Another bonus: Since they heat your entire body (not just your mouth), spicy foods speed up metabolism—so you won't gain as much.

Eat three squares *every* day. "A lot of people set themselves up for binges by restricting their food while dieting," says Dr. Scher. "When you skip breakfast and have nothing but a salad for lunch, by the time dinner rolls around, you're literally starving for food and will eat anything and everything. But if you consume three sensible meals each day—even while dieting—your body won't experience this intense starvation, and you'll be better able to control nighttime binges."

BREASTFEEDING

To your baby, your breasts are much more than a meal ticket. Study after study has shown that breastfed babies consistently seem to fare better than their formula-fed counterparts. In later years, they may score higher on IQ tests, and they're more immune to a host of problems ranging from diaper rash to cancer.

While mother's milk seems to offer Junior a smorgasbord of benefits, it isn't always a picnic to you: When you're nursing, your breasts may get hard and heavy, achy and swollen. Your nipples may feel more than a little bit chewed up. But if you want Junior to have the benefits, you probably want to go on breastfeeding. So here are some remedies to make the whole process smoother.

Eat garlic. Breast pain aside, perhaps the hardest part of breastfeeding is trying to convince the little tyke to eat well; some babies gnaw, bite and "play" with nipples, and they may not ingest enough milk for a good meal.

Researchers at the Monell Chemical Senses Center in Philadelphia found that mothers who eat 1.5 grams of garlic extract two hours before nursing got an odor in their milk that prompted infants to suck longer and possibly ingest more milk. Besides that, the babies experienced *no* abdominal cramps or other problems associated with spicy foods. If straight garlic isn't your idea of a tasty snack, try eating garlicky dishes before nursing.

Reposition your baby. The key to problem-free feeding is positioning. "The baby should face you entirely: head, chest, genitals, knees," suggests Marsha Walker, R.N., an international board-certified lactation consultant who is president of Lactation Associates in Weston, Massachusetts. According to Walker, you should grip the baby so that his buttocks are in one hand and his head is in the bend of your elbow. Let your other hand slip under your breast, with all four fingers supporting it. But don't put your fingers on the areola (the darker area around the nipple). Then tickle the baby's lower lip with your nipple to get his mouth open wide. When his mouth opens, pull his body in quickly so that his mouth fixes on the areola.

Go for depth. The nipple should be deep in the baby's throat, adds Carolyn Rawlins, M.D., an obstetrician in Munster, Indiana, and a member of the board of directors of La Leche League International, a support group for breastfeeding mothers, in Franklin Park, Illinois. "This way, there is no movement of the nipple when the baby sucks."

Use *both* breasts. Nurse on one side until it appears that the baby is losing interest, advises Walker. Then offer your baby the other side. Next time you feed, start with the side you ended with the time before. Some babies—especially newborns—won't take both breasts at one feeding, so Walker advises you offer the other side after about an hour, when the baby rouses a little.

Nurse often. "For women, there's often shock at how often a baby wants to nurse. Most doctors give instructions more appropriate to bottle feeding," says Julie Stock, medical information liaison for La Leche League International. You'll probably find yourself nursing 8 to 12 times a day in the early weeks.

Human milk was designed so that a baby needs to nurse frequently, says Dr. Rawlins. That creates better bonding between mother and child.

Say *ahhhh* with vitamin E. To soothe cracked nipples associated with breastfeeding, break open a vitamin E capsule and rub a small amount of the liquid on your nipples, advises Dr. Rawlins. The secret, however, is to use only a drop or two—and only apply it after you've finished nursing.

Or soothe with your own milk. Another effective treatment for hurting nipples is to express a little bit of milk and rub it in. Milk left at the end of the feeding is very high in lubricants and contains an antibiotic substance, says Dr. Rawlins.

CHOOSE A GOOD NURSING BRA

The best way to pick out a nursing bra is to go a cup size larger and a bra size bigger than your pregnancy bra, says Julie Stock of La Leche League International. "I wouldn't over-buy bras in the beginning. It's best to wait and see. By the third or fourth day, you may be able to wear your pregnancy bras."

Here are other tips for selecting a good bra.

- Choose all cotton over nylon.
- Make sure that the opening for nursing is wide enough so it doesn't compress the breast. That could lead to clogged ducts.
- Make sure you can easily open and close the bra with one hand. That will aid discretion.
- Avoid Velcro closings on the flaps because they make too much noise.
- Make sure the straps are comfortable and the bra isn't tight across the chest.

Stay alert to plugged ducts. Milk ducts can clog as a result of binding clothes, the mother's anatomy, fatigue or prolonged periods without nursing. A plugged duct can also signal the start of an infection if not dealt with promptly.

"If you feel a hard, painful-to-touch spot anywhere on the breast, get rid of it by using warmth," says Stock. Massage the breast, starting at the chest wall and working your way down with a circular motion.

Most important, however, allow your baby to nurse on that side frequently, she says. "Baby's sucking will help clear out that duct faster than anything else. Usually within 24 hours, it will be cleared up. The plug may be clear before you have physical evidence it's gone."

Try hot compresses to help with overproduction. If the baby is not keeping up with what mother is producing and

WHEN TO WEAN

How long should you nurse? "As long as you want to," says international lactation consultant Marsha Walker, R.N., of Massachusetts. In some societies, babies aren't weaned until they're 3 or 4. "The norm is well into the second year. That's traditional," says Walker.

Weaning, she says, "is appropriate when the baby or mother says it's enough. A lot of times it coincides with a developmental milestone like walking. The baby thinks, 'Do I want to walk more than I want the breast?' They cruise by and take a sip and run off. The mother may get tired of getting up four or five times a night or the baby moves onto other things."

Walker recommends that you wean gradually, stopping one or two feedings every few days and substituting cuddling, attention or playing. This way the baby isn't deprived of the closeness you and he have come to know as well as of the breast. You don't want to deprive yourself of the closeness, either.

you are getting overly full, put some hot, wet compresses on the breast, says Kittie Frantz, R.N., director of the Breast-Feeding Infant Clinic at the University of Southern California Medical Center in Los Angeles. It will open the ducts so the milk flows more freely.

Keep nipples from drying out. That means *no* soap on your nipples when you're showering, cautions Dr. Rawlins. "Do you see the little bumps around the areola? Those are glands that produce oil with natural antiseptic in it. So you don't need to use soap."

And after your shower, to prevent irritation, don't towel nipples dry; let them air-dry.

BREAST TENDERNESS

Diet, nutrition, water, weight, time of life, time of the month and hormones—some combination of these factors is likely to lead to breast tenderness some time in a woman's life. In fact, nearly three in four women suffer from breast pain and discomfort at least once in their adult lives. And some have this problem quite frequently.

Want relief?

Eat less meat. "The more animal proteins you eat, the slower your body will excrete estrogen," says Susan Doughty, R.N., a nurse practitioner at Women to Women, a clinic in Yarmouth, Maine. This excess estrogen often winds up in breast tissue, which is particularly sensitive to hormones.

Dehydrogenate your menu. Besides reducing meat and poultry, eliminate or drastically cut back on your intake of margarine and other hydrogenated fats, advises Christiane Northrup, M.D., assistant clinical professor of obstetrics and gynecology at the University of Vermont College of Medicine in Burlington. Hydrogenated fats interfere with your body's ability to convert essential fatty acids from the diet into gamma linoleic acid (GLA). Since your body needs GLA to help prevent breast pain, you may be asking for discomfort if you overdo hydrogenated fats and suppress the production of GLA.

Eliminate caffeine. The role of caffeine in contributing to breast discomfort has not been proven, but many doctors recommend no caffeine anyway. "I've seen women with pain and other symptoms of benign breast changes get markedly better after abstaining from caffeine," says Thomas J. Smith, M.D., director of the Breast Health Center at New England Medical Center in Boston. But you have to cut it *out*, not just *down*. Besides coffee and tea, other caffeinated items include soft drinks, chocolate, ice cream products and many over-the-counter pain relievers.

Get your vitamins. A good multivitamin/mineral supplement and a diet with plenty of foods rich in calcium, magnesium, vitamin C and B-complex vitamins are effective weapons against breast tenderness. Most of these vitamins indirectly affect the production of a hormone that can cause breast pain, says Dr. Northrup. Another helpful nutrient is vitamin E. "Many women find relief when they take a vitamin E supplement of 200 to 400 international units a day, particularly when they're experiencing pain," says Ellen Yankauskas, M.D., director of the Women's Center for Family Health in Atascadero, California.

Slim down if you need to. If you're overweight, simply dropping some of that excess weight may be enough to cure breast tenderness, says California nurse Kerry McGinn, R.N., author of *The Informed Woman's Guide to Breast Health.* In women, extra body fat makes the body produce more estrogen than the body needs.

Try these herbal teas. "Corn silk, buchu and uva ursi teas—available at most health food stores—are three very mild diuretics that seem to relieve breast tenderness in some women," says Dr. Yankauskas. By flushing fluid from your system, diuretics can help reduce breast swelling.

Or go the over-the-counter route. If you prefer to go with an over-the-counter pain reliever, look for one containing the active ingredient pamabron, Dr. Yankauskas advises. Pamabron acts as a mild diuretic.

BRITTLE NAILS

Trying to put a finger on the cause of frail nails? You could blame dry, overheated houses: When we stoke up the dry heat in winter, dry nails are one of the results. Or you could blame Father Time: After age 35, the natural aging process makes nails more brittle.

Mostly, though, you *should* blame water. "People don't realize that when your hands are soaking, your nails can absorb between 20 and 25 percent of their weight in water," says Herbert Luscombe, M.D., professor emeritus of dermatology at Jefferson Medical College of Thomas Jefferson University in Philadelphia and senior attending dermatologist at Thomas Jefferson University Hospital. "So if you do a lot of dishes, or swimming, or even bathing, you're more prone to brittle nails."

Nails expand as they absorb water, then contract when hands are dry. The more water you expose nails to, the more they expand and contract—and that weakens them. But here's how to keep them firm, so they're tough enough to withstand the rigors of clean living and water sports.

Chow down on cauliflower. A little-known nutrient called biotin can thicken nails to help prevent splitting and cracking. "Biotin is absorbed into the core of the nail, where it may encourage a better, thicker nail to grow," says Richard K. Scher, M.D., professor of dermatology and head of the Nail Section at Columbia University–Presbyterian Medical Center in New York City. Cauliflower is a rich source of biotin, as are legumes such as peanuts and lentils. One study showed that people consuming 2,500 micrograms (2.5 milligrams) of biotin daily had marked increases in nail thickness after six months. To get this much biotin, you'll need to take it in supplement form.

Get cookin' with cooking oil. "A regular soaking with vegetable oil is very effective. It replenishes the moisture lost from having your hands in and out of water frequently," says Dr. Luscombe. In fact, vegetable oils *are* better than many commercially sold nail care products because they don't have the alcohol-containing fragrances that can dry out nails.

Messy soaking in oil isn't necessary: Just brush on the oil and massage it into the nail. "I put some safflower or vegetable oil in a clean, empty nail polish bottle and brush it on my nails several times a day," says hand model Trisha Webster, who works for the Wilhelmina Modeling Agency in New York City. "And don't forget to put a drop of oil on the underside of the nail at your fingertip."

Use an over-the-counter moisturizer. You should moisturize nails right after you wash your hands. "And do it every time," says Paul Kechijian, M.D., clinical associate professor of dermatology and chief of the Nail Section at New York University Medical Center in New York City. If you use a commercial moisturizer, look for the kind that contains urea or lactic acid, two ingredients that attract and bind moisture to your nails.

Trim nails short. If you're plagued by brittle nails, trim them shorter, advises Dr. Kechijian. Longer nails are just more likely to crack or tear. Trim your nails right after washing or bathing, when they're softer and less likely to crack or break.

Massage your fingertips. "Regularly massage your fingertips to improve blood circulation around your nails," says Webster. She suggests three or four times a day—or at least in the morning and evening. If you use some petroleum jelly while you're at it, you'll moisturize as you massage.

Don't play taps. Forget that old folk remedy that calls for tapping your nails on a hard surface in order to toughen them. "If you traumatize them in some way, they *will* grow faster," says Dr. Scher. "And because they are newer, younger nails, they may seem like they are stronger, but they're really not." For the same reason, avoid nail biting: Your nervous nibbling is just another trauma for your nails.

THUMBNAILS DOWN ON STRENGTHENERS

Nail strengtheners may be touted as the way to turn weak and brittle nails into unbreakables. In reality, most claims for these products are excessive, according to Richard K. Scher, M.D., professor of dermatology and head of the Nail Section at Columbia University–Presbyterian Medical Center in New York City.

Nail strengtheners supposedly contain an ingredient that binds to damaged nails and makes them thicker. But you can't change the nail structure by applying something to the surface, says Paul Kechijian, M.D., clinical associate professor of dermatology and chief of the Nail Section at New York University Medical Center in New York City. "At best, nail strengtheners protect the nail plate, so they won't peel," he says. "They merely camouflage the brittleness."

Glove 'em if you love 'em. Washing dishes? *"Always* wear rubber gloves with separate cotton gloves inside," says Dr. Kechijian. "The rubber keeps water off your nails, and the cotton absorbs sweat, so nails won't get soggy *inside* the gloves."

He suggests keeping a half-dozen pairs of cotton gloves on hand and washing and drying them after each use. That way, you'll always have a clean, dry pair each time you do the dishes.

CELLULITE

Cellulite is actually no more than pockets of fat, says Paul Lazar, M.D., professor of clinical dermatology at Northwestern University Medical School. Its appearance is due to strands of fibrous tissue anchored to the skin, pulling the skin inward and, in the process, plumping the fat cells outward. Some people may be more susceptible to cellulite than others, Dr. Lazar says—especially women, who generally are more fatty and less muscular in the buttocks, hips, and thighs than men.

Some nonmedical skin specialists see cellulite as more than just fat. "Cellulite is a combination of fat globules, waste matter and water imprisoned in connective tissue," says Carole Walderman, aesthetician and president of Von Lee International School of Aesthetics, in Baltimore.

Medical doctors and researchers may not agree with this theory. Neither are they likely to agree that much can be done to get rid of cellulite once it sets in. Cellulite is something you can try to avoid, says Dr. Lazar, through exercise and by keeping your weight normal. But those face-to-face with cellulite are willing to give *something* a try. We weeded through the claims, tossed out the bizarre and came up with the following middle-of-the-road remedies. They're yours for the trying.

Peel off the pounds. Since cellulite is fat, excess weight can contribute to it, says Dr. Lazar. Lose weight gradually, he says, and "hopefully, some of what you lose will be cellulite."

Eat plenty of fresh fruit and vegetables—low in calories yet packed with nutrients—and drink fruit and vegetable juices, suggests Dolores Schneider, a nutritionist and director of Sharon Springs, a spa in upstate New York where people go to lose pounds and detoxify their bodies.

Get back in balance by eating well. Eat a healthy, balanced diet overall, urges Kim Ulen, supervisor of the skin care department of the Cal-a-Vie Spa in Vista, California. "This returns your body chemistry to a balanced state in which cellulite is less likely to develop," she says.

Get back in balance by resting well. Relax in your bathtub, Schneider suggests, with a home mineral bath containing sea salt. Add about 2 cups of sea salt to warm bathwater and luxuriate in the soothing waters for at least 20 minutes. It will leave your skin feeling smooth.

Combat constipation. "People who are constipated on a regular basis usually have cellulite," says Ulen. Your meals move more quickly through your digestive tract when you eat plenty of high-fiber foods like green vegetables and grains every day, she says. For an extra boost, she suggests sprinkling raw bran on your foods or in your beverages at each meal.

Make your skin an exit ramp. According to skin specialists, keeping your body's natural highways and byways clear gives cellulite an easier escape route. To open up the blood vessels in and just below your skin, and also to keep your waste-removal system working properly, drink lots of water and steer clear of salt, coffee and cigarettes, which constrict your blood vessels and may actually make your cellulite more prominent.

Take up muscle-toning exercises. Building stronger muscles with methods such as Nautilus or working out with weights may help fill out the tissue in cellulite problem areas, says Dr. Lazar.

Massage those trouble spots. Reinforce the benefits of exercise, says Ulen, with gentle, kneading massage you can do yourself in areas like your thighs and the insides of your knees.

Take a deep breath. Learn to breathe from deep down in your diaphragm, says Schneider. The oxygen helps burn fat. A deep breath also helps clean out toxic carbon dioxide from all your cells, says Ulen.

CERVICAL DYSPLASIA

The last word any woman wants to hear following a Pap smear is "abnormal." It is not, however, a reason for panic. "Abnormal" findings are extremely common and are usually due to easy-to-treat conditions such as inflammation, an infection or cervical erosion. It's also possible to learn that you have what doctors call cervical dysplasia.

This condition often causes no symptoms—it's simply the growth of abnormal cells on the cervix. (The cervix, located deep within the vagina, is the opening to the uterus.) But because some kinds of cervical dysplasia set the stage for the development of cervical cancer, doctors often treat cervical dysplasia aggressively, removing the cells in moderate or severe cases and, in mild cases, either removing cells or monitoring them closely with frequent Pap smears. (The cells may revert to normal or become increasingly abnormal.)

PROTECTING YOURSELF

Unlike heart disease or lung cancer, cervical cancer—and its precursor, cervical dysplasia—isn't generally thought of as a "lifestyle" disease. But population studies do link an increased risk for cervical cancer with some factors that are within your control. Following these tips will help you reduce your risk.

Get regular Pap smears. "The biggest risk factor for invasive cervical cancer is infrequent Pap smears," says Ruth Peters, Sc.D., a professor of preventive medicine at the University of Southern California School of Medicine in Los Angeles.

Most experts recommend that you begin getting Pap smears as soon as you become sexually active. After you've had *three* consecutive annual Pap smears that show all is normal, you shouldn't need another for three more years. If the test shows that something cancerous may be brewing, more frequent testing is highly advisable, says Dr. Peters.

One study by researchers at the University of Washington found that women who hadn't had a Pap test in ten years or more had *12 times* the cancer risk of women who got checked more regularly.

Make it monogamous. The more sexual partners you've had, the higher your risk for cervical cancer. And if you're faithful but he's been sleeping around, your risks also shoot up. Why? Chances are you, through your mate, have been exposed to a virus associated with cervical cancer. "Strains of human papillomavirus (HPV) have been found in more than 90 percent of cervical cancer tissue samples," says Ralph Richart, M.D., director of the Division of Gynecological Pathology and Cytology at Columbia Presbyterian Medical Center in New York City.

Wait till you're twentysomething. Because it may expose cervical cells to the sexually transmitted factor (perhaps HPV) at a time when they are particularly vulnerable, sex at an early age ups your risk for developing cervical cancer later, Dr. Peters says. "In one recent study, one partner before age 20 tripled a woman's risk, and three or more sexual partners before age 20 increased the risk tenfold," she says.

Use barrier methods of birth control. Condoms and diaphragms protect the cervix from contact with lots of potential irritants, including the HPV virus. In her study, Dr. Peters also found contraceptive creams, jellies and foams reduced cancer risks. Why? "They kill sperm, and they probably also kill whatever else might be transmitted," she says.

Douche with discretion. Don't douche unless your doctor tells you to. There is a misperception among many women that regular douching keeps you fresh and clean. Instead, it seems to reduce the body's natural ability to fight off disease. "In one recent study, douching five or more times a month tripled the risk of cervical cancer," says Dr. Peters

Ditch your butts, and his, too. Studies show that smoking triples your risk for cervical cancer, Dr. Peters says. "Nicotine and other chemicals from cigarette smoke are concentrated in the cervical fluid," she says. Those same toxins also end up in a man's semen.

One study showed that women exposed to passive cigarette smoke for three or more hours a day had a threefold increase in cervical cancer.

Eat better. Numerous population studies have linked the development of cervical cancer with poor nutrition. Adequate intake of vitamins E and C, beta-carotene and folate seems protective.

GET PROPER TREATMENT

What do you need to know if you are told you have cervical dysplasia? In a sense, you should be delighted that your doctor has found these abnormal cells. Early treatment can prevent them from turning into cancer.

Next you should be aware that your diagnosis should not be based on a Pap smear alone. "A Pap smear is a screening test, not a method of diagnosis," says Robert Kurman, M.D., a professor and director of gynecologic pathology at Johns Hopkins Hospital in Baltimore.

An abnormal Pap smear indicating dysplasia should be followed by a biopsy of the cervix done with a colposcope, a viewing instrument that provides a magnified view of the cervix and allows the doctor to see any actual lesions, Dr. Kurman says. The biopsy removes small bits of tissue that are examined under a microscope. At the same time, the doctor may also scrape cells from the opening to the uterus, a procedure called endocervical curettage. Based on the examination of these two tissue samples, the doctor will decide how much cervical tissue needs to be removed and how it should be removed.

The tissue is most often removed by freezing (cryosurgery) or carbon dioxide laser surgery, both simple outpatient procedures. If the abnormal cells have invaded underlying tissue, a more radical surgical procedure, or radiation therapy, may be required.

A newer technique that uses a thin, electrically charged wire loop to scoop out areas of abnormal cells may be better than ei-

SYMPTOMS THAT SAY SEE YOUR DOCTOR

Ideally, a woman should have her first pelvic examination by about age 18 or when she becomes sexually active—whichever comes first.

After that, many doctors, including Cornell University Medical College's Yvonne S. Thornton, M.D., recommend one every year.

But preventive care isn't the only reason you should see your gynecologist. A trip to the doctor is also warranted for the following female reproductive system symptoms.

- If you haven't begun menstruating by age 16.
- If your mother took the now-banned drug diethylstilbestrol (DES), once used to help problem pregnancies come to full term. Daughters of DES mothers have been found to be at an increased risk for uterine and cervical cancers.
- If you've been suffering from severe menstrual cramps.
- If your menstrual flow is very heavy or lasts longer than ten days or you experience any other vaginal bleeding.
- If you experience any burning, itching or unusual discharge.
- If you've been experiencing painful intercourse, especially if you also have chills or fever.
- If you are sexually active and have missed one period.
- If you miss three or more periods and are abstaining from sex.
- Any time you have burning when you urinate.

ther cryosurgery or laser surgery, though, Dr. Richart says. "The procedure is easy to teach and learn," he says. "It requires less expensive equipment than other methods of removal, allows biopsy and treatment to occur at the same time, which saves patients an additional office visit, and gives a complete tissue sample for examination, which will do away with missed diagnosis of invasive cancer."

CONCEPTION PROBLEMS

The one thing that can be more frustrating than being a parent is trying to become one with no success. For one in seven couples, conceiving a child can be a long and difficult process—it can take at least one year and sometimes requires several.

Some "trying" couples are infertile because of physical problems. But most couples are simply "underfertile"—they are physically able to conceive but have to nudge the stork just a bit more than usual. Here's what experts recommend for them.

Take cough syrup. "Before we had high-tech measures, a lot of doctors would recommend that women take cough syrup containing guaifenesin about four times a day around the time of ovulation," says Arthur L. Wisot, M.D., a fertility specialist who is affiliated with the Center for Advanced Reproductive Care in Redondo Beach, California. "And that's still sound advice, because guaifenesin thins the cervical mucus, making it easier for sperm to swim through to meet the egg."

Don't lubricate with commercial products. When intercourse needs a helping hand, couples sometimes use a commercial lubricant like K-Y jelly. But that can hurt your chances of conceiving. That's because these products can impair sperm, making them less able to reach the egg, says John Willems, M.D., associate clinical professor of obstetrics and gynecology at the University of California, San Diego, and a researcher at the Scripps Clinic and Research Foundation in La Jolla. "A woman's natural lubricants should be all you need."

But egg white may help. If you need a lubricant during intercourse, try using egg white instead of a pharmaceutical lubricant, suggests Andrew Toledo, M.D., a fertility specialist and reproductive endocrinologist who is assistant clinical professor of medicine in the Department of Gynecology and Obstetrics at Emory University in Atlanta. Because the egg white lubricant is pure protein—as is sperm—it makes a better "carrier" than lubricants made from nonprotein substances.

If dryness is a problem, Dr. Toledo recommends using the egg white lubricant during the days when a woman is fertile and a regular lubricant the rest of the time. But don't use egg white if you're allergic to it, and be sure to separate the white from the yolk before applying it to either the penis or the vagina.

Take more vitamin C. Studies by researchers at the University of Texas Medical Branch at Galveston show that large doses of vitamin C can *reverse* some cases of male infertility. The team there, headed by Earl B. Dawson, Ph.D., reported that men who increased their vitamin C intake to 1,000 milligrams daily (the Recommended Dietary Allowance is 60 milligrams) showed increased sperm count, motility and longevity.

Stub out cigarettes. Smokers' alert: Women who smoke have more difficulty getting pregnant, according to studies by researchers at the National Institute of Environmental Health Sciences in Research Triangle Park, North Carolina. "But we don't yet understand the biological reason why," says Allen Wilcox, M.D., Ph.D., chief of the Epidemiology Branch at the institute. So if you smoke, you may better your chances of conception by giving it up.

Practice clean living. Smoking isn't the only vice that hurts your chances of conceiving. Studies at the National Institute of Environmental Health Sciences showed that women who drink just one cup of coffee daily may halve their chances of becoming pregnant each menstrual cycle (compared with those who don't get any caffeine). "Cutting out caffeine seems to help some women, but not others. It may be worth a try," says Dr. Wilcox.

And there are other factors to consider as well. "You need to get your act together—don't use drugs, stop drinking and avoid all unnecessary medications," says Dr. Wisot. He also recommends that women start taking prenatal vitamins.

Wear boxer shorts. For some men, fashionable underwear styles may be the shortcut to fatherhood. Tight-fitting jockey shorts pull the testicles close to the body, and body heat impairs sperm, according to Dr. Wisot. He recommends wearing looser-fitting boxer shorts.

Don't soak in a hot tub, guys. High-temperature water can also lower sperm count and motility, says Dr. Wisot, so the man who wants to be Dad should stay away from hot tubs.

Go missionary. Although sexual position usually has no bearing on conception, "the missionary position assures better contact of the semen with the cervix—and may make the difference in marginal cases," says Dr. Wisot.

Keep a calendar. Most fertility specialists say that you and your partner should try to conceive for at least one year before assuming you have a conception problem.

"Generally, if a woman has an average 28-day cycle, she will begin ovulating on the 14th day," says Dr. Wisot. "If she's on an irregular cycle, ovulation usually occurs 14 days before her next expected menstrual cycle." Keeping track on a calendar for a few months is a good way to see your pattern.

Get help from a kit. "There are several ovulation kits that you can buy over the counter that help tell a woman when she's ovulating," adds Dr. Wisot. "Starting on the 16th or 17th day before your period, you should test your urine each evening with these kits. When you get a positive test, have intercourse the next day."

Go for the gold the second time around. Probably the biggest mistake couples make is assuming that a man's first ejaculation is his best. Actually, a woman is more likely to get pregnant when a man ejaculates two days before she starts ovulation and then they wait until she is ovulating before they try to conceive. "Usually that second specimen is better, both in sperm count and motility," says Dr. Wisot.

DIETING

osing weight is such a way of life among American women, dieting is considered "normal" eating. In fact, some researchers have found so much in common between dieters and women with eating disorders, they have come to see anorexia and bulimia as simply "the extreme end of the continuum" of female eating behavior, according to Kathleen Pike, Ph.D., a psychologist who studies and treats eating disorders at the New York Psychiatric Institute at Columbia Presbyterian Medical Center.

Many dieters have the same skewed body image as people with eating disorders, seeing fat where others see slimness. If you are not one yourself, you know a chronic dieter. She may have 5 or 10 or 20 pounds to lose—or none at all. But for all the blood, sweat and tears (and occasionally, pounds) she sheds dieting, it might as well be 100.

Many dieters suffer from what therapist Kim Chernin, author of *The Obsession: Reflections on the Tyranny of Slenderness*, calls pseudo-obesity. At or near their ideal weight, they are nevertheless driven "toward a condition of ruddy-cheeked emaciation" idealized by models and actresses who are unusually tall and thin.

Like anorexics and bulimics, chronic dieters are always dieting, yet thinking, dreaming, obsessing about food.

FEELING FAT

Not surprisingly, chronic dieters are almost always women. "For an overwhelming number of women in our society, being a woman means feeling too fat," write Yale University researchers Judith Rodin, Ph.D., Lisa Silberstein and Ruth Striegel-Moore, who have explored some of the pressures on women to "pursue thinness like a career."

For women, the heat is on by the time they're 9. A study done by a University of California researcher of 494 girls between 9 and 18 found that an astonishing number—31 percent—were already binge eating by age 9, with another third admitting they were afraid of getting fat. By the time those girls reach college, according to another study, more than half are engaging in unhealthful dietary practices, such as bingeing and vomiting. And it apparently never ends. In a study on elderly women conducted by Dr. Rodin and her colleagues at Yale, their greatest personal concern, next to memory loss, was their weight.

WHERE IT BEGINS

There was a time, not so long ago, when abundant flesh was considered sexy. And we're not harking back to the round and rosy nudes of the painter Rubens. In the 1950s, the ultraslim, ultrasleek Audrey Hepburn was considered beautiful and glamorous, but it was Marilyn Monroe who had sex appeal.

Today, there are millions of women who were raised on the images of virtual 98-pound weaklings, like 1960s supermodel Twiggy, whose figures were decidedly boyish—or prepubescent girlish—and strikingly like the cadaverous silhouettes of anorexics whose disorder some researchers see as a backlash against maturation and womanhood. In fact, several researchers have suggested that the quest for thinness is an expression of sexual liberation, since a thin body represents athleticism and androgyny—if not downright masculinity—rather than motherliness.

There are other reasons, too. Fat is considered unhealthy and has been associated with a variety of ailments, including heart disease. Studies have also shown that even as children, we think of fat as "bad," a virtual moral transgression. Fat people are so stigmatized that we regard overweight with almost as much dread as mortal illness. In one telling study when children with juvenile diabetes were asked if they would trade their life-threatening disease for obesity, most said no.

Unfortunately for most women, attractiveness is currency. It's what buys acceptance, the best man, the best job, the best life. With few exceptions, most people don't consider a fat woman beautiful.

OUR BODIES, OUR SELVES

Why do ordinary women aspire to the angularity of, say, model Paulina or actress Julia Roberts, whose bodies are tools of their trade and who have body sizes natural to only about 5 percent of the population?

For most women, genetics makes the attainment of that particular body type nearly impossible. And therein lies the rub. Our culture, says social historian Roberta Pollack Seid in her book *Never Too Thin*, "has set up a female body standard that is antithetical to female biology." Although we may resist the idea that biology is destiny, when it comes to our bodies, it is. A woman needs a fat-to-lean ratio of about 22 percent to start and maintain menstruation. Under that figure, we risk bone-thinning amenorrhea (an absence of the menstrual cycle) and infertility.

We are also circumscribed by what some diet experts call our setpoints, the weight we can maintain without conscious effort. When we go below our setpoint weight, our bodies seek the former status quo, conserving energy and boosting our appetites, one of the major reasons dieting is nearly always a losing battle.

DIETING IS BAD FOR YOUR HEALTH

There are other reasons to jump off the dieting treadmill. For one, chronic dieting is a form of malnutrition. It's not healthy. "Losing weight can be as harmful as overweight, with an impressive array of health hazards accompanying it," according to eating disorders researchers Janet Polivy, Ph.D., and Linda Thomsen. Although overweight can be a serious health problem for certain people, notably those with high blood pressure and diabetes, there is evidence that for most people the dangers have been overestimated. Some researchers believe that being moderately obese—up to 25 percent above standard body weight—doesn't affect long-term health.

There's also evidence that dieting—particularly very-low-calorie or bizarre diet plans—can *cause* a variety of ailments including gallstones, headaches, nausea, muscle aches, fatigue, anemia, cardiac disorders and even death in rare cases. You can feel tired and unable to concentrate even on a balanced diet. Studies, including the famous Framingham Heart Study, have found that so-called yo-yo dieting may shift body fat to the abdominal area, where fat is associated with more diabetes, high blood pressure and heart disease.

HOW TO BE A HAPPY LOSER

What if you really need to lose weight? How do you shed the lose/gain, lose/gain syndrome and end up a winner at losing?

"Any diet that works is going to have to teach you new eating habits you can carry out for the rest of your life," says New York psychologist and eating disorder expert Kathleen Pike, Ph.D. "As soon as you begin thinking you're going to be on a diet for six weeks and then the diet is over, you are set up to gain weight again. People say they go to diet programs because 'I don't have to think about it. I just open the box and eat it.' The problem is that in order for it to work long term, you have to think about it."

One relatively painless way to lose weight is to stop counting calories and begin counting fat. In a 22-week study at Cornell University, 13 women who ate a low-fat diet (getting 25 percent of their calories from fat) without restricting how many calories or how much food they ate, lost weight slowly for months without having to give up any goodies. They could eat pizza, ice cream and cookies, as long as they were low in fat.

Researchers estimate you can lose 10 percent of your body weight in a year just by cutting back on fat.

And you have to exercise. Exercise, along with firming and building muscles and burning calories, is what allows you to eat more. You can burn roughly 200 calories or more, depending on your weight, just by taking a brisk (3½ miles per hour) half-hour walk every day. It can mean the difference between listening to your stomach growl on 1,000 calories a day and feeding it a couple of snacks to tide it over at 1,200 calories a day.

In fact, researchers have found that the difference between long-time weight losers and those who gain it back is exercise, as little as 3.3 hours of it a week, according to one expert.

Just be wary of taking exercise to the same extremes that many take dieting.

DIETING MAKES YOU FAT

There are psychological hazards as well. Many dieters may recognize what experts call the dieting depression syndrome as those feelings of irritability, anxiety, depression, apathy, mood swings and fatigue that accompany all those carrot sticks and 8-ounce glasses of water.

Dieters may also be oversensitive to stress and turn to eating to relieve it. Not only do they find comfort in eating, but many choose sugar-laden, high-carbohydrate foods, which research has found increase mood-elevating chemicals in the brain—the Twinkie as a natural high. In fact, a number of studies have found that dieting can lead to binge eating, which may account for why so many dieters who "took it all off" put it all back on again. In other words, dieting can *make* you fat.

"When you go on high-restraint diets that essentially are unsustainable, you set yourself up to binge or eat compulsively," explains Dr. Pike. "Once you get into that cycle—restraint then bingeing—ultimately the restraint loses and the eating wins out."

You become the victim of "weight cycling." Once you stop your diet, your body goes into famine-survival mode. Your metabolism is slowed down and your body has become more efficient at storing fat. If you go back to your old eating habits—hunger is such a primal urge, most people do—you often find yourself weighing more than you did when you first started. You can diet again, says Dr. Pike, "but your body has become so efficient you don't lose as much weight."

How do you know if you need to diet or are simply a victim of the current quest for ultrathinness? You need to do a reality check, says Dr. Pike. Ask people you know and trust—a friend, your doctor or nurse—if they think you need to lose weight. Some studies have found that many women—95 percent in one research project—overestimate the size of their bodies more as a result of how they feel about themselves than of how they see themselves.

You may also be doing some "magical" thinking, says Dr. Pike. Many women believe that thinness equals happiness. "Sometimes a certain weight is associated with a happy time when you were

COMFORT FOODS

For most of us, food isn't just food. It's everything from love to medicine. It's stimulating and soothing, comforting and calming. "To say food is just to sustain life," says California psychologist Joyce Nash, Ph.D., author of *Maximize Your Body Potential,* "is like saying sex is only for procreation."

For some women, food satiates many hungers. Recent studies have found that people who have been traumatized as children—who were sexually abused, neglected or lost a parent—may use food for comfort and nurturing. "As children, when they didn't know how to cope with their feelings, they did something that felt good, that helped them cope, and they maintain those bad habits long after," says Ronette Kolotkin, Ph.D., clinical psychologist at the Duke University Diet and Fitness Center in Durham, North Carolina.

Food can "provide a distraction from whatever problems really exist," says Dr. Nash. For many women, food serves as an escape, a way to avoid or cope with their problems.

that weight. You think, 'If I go back to that weight, I will achieve that level of happiness.' Often women believe there is some kind of cause and effect, that reaching a certain weight will guarantee them all kinds of happiness and pleasure."

Comforting—or distressing—as it might be to think, "If I lost 20 pounds, I'd be happy," the truth is you will still be you. The thin person inside every fat person is the same person without cellulite.

EARLOBE PAIN

Your new silver earrings with copper inlays were *perfect* with that outfit. And even though they made your earlobes itch after a couple of hours, you kept on wearing them for a couple more! So today you're gingerly fingering two tender, red, weeping earlobes.

Blame your angry earlobes on nickel, which is in virtually *all* jewelry. One in ten women is allergic or sensitive to this common metal, says William Epstein, M.D., professor of dermatology at the University of California, San Francisco, School of Medicine. But if you notice the reaction—known as dermatitis—and treat it before mere inflammation becomes real infection, you can easily do a favor for your inflamed earlobes.

Remove your earrings. You won't "build up resistance" to the nickel that's causing your skin to rebel—so once you've taken off the offending earrings, keep them off. "Once you're allergic to something, assume you're always going to be allergic to it," says Hillard H. Pearlstein, M.D., assistant clinical professor of dermatology at Mount Sinai School of Medicine in New York City.

Try a lobe bath. Clean your lobes with hydrogen peroxide, says Nancy Sculerati, M.D., assistant professor of otolaryngology and director of pediatric otolaryngology at New York University Medical Center in New York City. Mix equal parts peroxide and water. (Rubbing alcohol also works, but it tends to sting, she says.) Pour the solution over the earlobe, or apply it with gauze, and let the runoff drip into a sink. Don't apply the liquid with cotton balls if the ear is weepy, says Dr. Sculerati, because the cotton will stick to the earlobe.

Stop the itch. To soothe itchy rashes that are oozing or weeping, use Domeboro powder, which you can get in a drugstore, suggests D'Anne Kleinsmith, M.D., a cosmetic dermatologist with William Beaumont Hospital near Detroit. Mix the powder with water at *half* the recommended strength, says Dr. Kleinsmith.

Dip a washcloth or gauze pad in the solution and hold it on the ear for a minute or so. Let the ear dry, then repeat once. This will have a "drawing" effect on the earlobe and will help dry up the dermatitis, says Dr. Kleinsmith.

Recommended frequency: Use the compresses three times a day at first, then taper off treatment during the next three or four days. As soon as the oozing or crusting stops, stop using the compresses, Dr. Kleinsmith says, or you'll dry your skin too much.

Fight the itch with cream. Mild dermatitis might meet its match if you fight it with 1 percent hydrocortisone cream, available without prescription at most drugstores. Dr. Epstein suggests applying some cream directly to the earlobes, following the package directions. If this doesn't help, he says you may need a prescription for a stronger steroid treatment.

Keep both hands on the table. "Pay attention to your hands," Dr. Epstein suggests. If you pick or pull at your irritated earlobes, the dermatitis could worsen into a low-grade infection, he says. You'll know it's on its way when the earlobe thickens or becomes sore.

Apply antibiotics. For mild, superficial infections, limited to a tiny earlobe area, you can buy Neosporin or Polysporin antibiotic ointment, says Kenneth H. Neldner, M.D., professor and chairman of the Department of Dermatology at Texas Tech University Health Sciences Center in Lubbock. Keep the earlobe clean with antibacterial soap, and use an antibiotic ointment two or three times a day, he says. The infection should go away in a few days. If it doesn't, see a dermatologist.

Keep those openings unclogged. If your earring holes become clogged with dry skin or oil, douse them once a day with a mild astringent such as Sea Breeze, witch hazel or alcohol, suggests Dr. Pearlstein. This will help prevent waxy, dried body oil (sebum) from coagulating in the holes.

EARS: A HIGH-RISK LOCATION

Ears are prone to sunburn because they stick out like wings on a plane," says Hillard H. Pearlstein, M.D., assistant clinical professor of dermatology at the Mount Sinai School of Medicine in New York City. "That's why they're extremely susceptible to cancerous change," he says. Any change in the texture or color of the skin on the ears warrants a trip to a dermatologist.

Also, small, hard lumps in the earlobes—called fibromas—are common, says William Epstein, M.D., professor of dermatology at the University of California, San Francisco, School of Medicine. A fibroma usually is not serious, but only a doctor can tell. "If one comes up where it hadn't been before, or if one grows, a doctor should look at it," he says.

Go for the gold. When your dermatitis has cleared up and you're ready to try on earrings again, buy high-grade gold or pure silver, suggests Dr. Neldner. One warning before you empty your bank account, however: There's no guarantee this will solve your problem, because even 18-karat gold contains nickel, says Dr. Pearlstein.

"You may be able to wear pearl, ceramic, glass or plastic earrings with gold posts or surgical steel posts and be just fine, though," says Dr. Kleinsmith.

Coat them with polish. "You can try painting the backs of bothersome earrings with clear nail polish," suggests Dr. Kleinsmith. The lacquer creates a barrier between the metal and your skin. Use Almay or Clinique nail polish, which contains no formaldehyde, to reduce your chances of having a reaction to that common allergen, she says.

EATING DISORDERS

T hirty years ago Marilyn Monroe had the ideal shape: rounded and full of curves. "Yet if she were alive now and in her prime, she would be considered fat," says psychologist Robert Mann, Ph.D., vice president and clinical director of The Rader Institute, a nationwide eating disorder clinic with headquarters in Los Angeles. "Thirty years ago the 'ideal' figure was achievable. Not now." Every magazine cover and ad, movie and TV show reminds you of the modern "ideal" body: stick-slender, with a minute percentage of body fat that women are not physiologically destined to attain. Yet try to attain it they do—with fad diets, endless exercise and constant self-critiques in the mirror.

And some people take this body dissatisfaction to such an extreme that it becomes a mental illness—the eating disorders anorexia and bulimia, or a combination of both. "The anorexic sees in the mirror something that isn't there," Dr. Mann says. "She shows you her emaciated arms with bones and joints sticking out and says, 'Look how fat I am.'" To shed that imaginary fat, she starves herself. Most doctors label someone an anorexic who falls to 15 percent or more below her ideal body weight.

The bulimic, on the other hand, says, "I want to look like [insert the name of any currently popular, impossibly thin media star]." She typically cannot be found after dinner—where she's just binged on a king-size filet of beef, a baked potato smothered with butter and sour cream and three slices of ice cream-covered apple pie—unless you check the bathroom. There you'll find her forcing herself to vomit. Bingeing and purging—either by vomiting or with laxatives—are the classic symptoms of bulimia.

THE ROOTS OF EATING DISORDERS

Why do some people take the normal desire to look good and run amok with it? Some of the cause may lie in their family background, says psychiatrist Joel Yager, M.D., professor of psychiatry at the University of California, Los Angeles, and senior consultant in the UCLA Neuropsychiatric Institute's Adult Eating Disorders Program. "Their families often have higher levels of dysfunction," he says. "There's a higher alcoholism rate among the fathers, a higher rate of depression among the mothers. Often there's been a divorce or a chronically unhappy marriage. And physical abuse is common in these families—it has been reported by 86 percent of the patients that Dr. Mann sees in the hospital, admittedly a worst-case setting. Where some people choose drugs, promiscuity or other extremes to dull or forget their psychological pain, others choose food.

Ninety-five percent of people with eating disorders are women between the ages of 12 and 25. Some studies estimate that 4.5 percent of 18-year-old college women are bulimic, while the rate of anorexia is up to 1 percent in females 12 to 18 years old. One study of female professional tennis players revealed 30 percent of them were bulimic, Dr. Mann says. Ironically, he adds, "another huge bulimic population is student dietitians—one study indicated as high as 40 percent."

The starvation an anorexic imposes on herself can kill her. And a bulimic "does murderous things to her gastrointestinal system," Dr. Mann says.

Anorexia is the more dangerous of the two disorders. "Ten percent of anorexics die," Dr. Mann says. Malnourishment can be deadly. Their muscles atrophy and waste away. Their blood pressure drops to dangerous levels. Their periods stop. Abuse of laxatives causes dehydration. They have low resistance to infection. They develop potassium deficiencies, which can cause heart damage and heart attacks. Others become depressed—depression that may be exacerbated by nutritional deficiencies.

But bulimics don't get off easy. "They can test anywhere from healthy to critically ill," Dr. Mann says. Repetitive vomiting lets stomach acid scar the esophagus and throat and erode tooth enamel. Some bulimics habitually take Ipecac, an over-the-counter drug that induces vomiting. "It's sometimes a testament to the resilience of the human body that a bulimic can maintain good health," he says. But he's not talking about good mental health—bulimics also often suffer depression.

Regardless of what led to your anorexia or bulimia, you can learn how to overcome it.

A VOTE FOR VOLUPTUOUS

Like any mental illness, anorexia or bulimia can leave you feeling hollow and alone. It's hard to see your way out. But there *is* a way out—and help can be tailored to fit you, says Robert Mann, Ph.D., of The Rader Institute, a nationwide eating disorder clinic. What you have to do is face the facts of your eating disorder, choose your treatment plan and learn how to eat right.

Serious cases of anorexia and bulimia have their roots far deeper than the superficial appeal of trying to look like the ideal woman, yet that false hope serves as the spur for all the physical and emotional torture anorexics and bulimics force themselves to endure.

Although we're all subject to society's whims of fashion and body size, the best thing you can do, experts say, is try for a more reasonable—and possibly more rounded—ideal.

Pick up the telephone. If you have bulimic tendencies, Dr. Yager says, understanding what's creating your problem will help in dealing with it. Learn all you can about the disease and consider joining an eating disorders group, where you can get counseling from professionals and those who've "been there."

Find a good confidant. "It's always good to tell somebody else 'I have this problem, and I'm going to try to get better,' because then you've made a statement and you feel you have to stick to it," Dr. Yager says.

Check out nutritional counseling. The most important thing you can do is get back on a sound eating program. Colleges—those hotbeds of bulimia where newly arrived freshmen begin copying the bingeing and purging traits of their dormitory peers—often offer education, peer counseling and student health programs.

Get professional help. Serious cases of bulimia, says Dr. Yager, require more than self-help. "Bulimia is more serious when it's accompanied by depression," Dr. Yager notes, "and if that's the case, the person is better off with professional help. Some depression is a response to bulimia that's out of control, but some bulimia is a symptom of depression." Antidepressants are sometimes prescribed.

Choosing a treatment plan. The surest cure for anorexia, says Dr. Yager, is through professional help. A professional program usually includes a nutritionist and a psychiatrist, sometimes a psychologist and your family doctor or pediatrician. If you're anorexic, says Dr. Yager, you may have some physical problems, and it's likely your laboratory tests may show all kinds of abnormalities. These have to be monitored closely, so it's likely you'll have to be hospitalized, at least for a while.

"The reason is that anorexics are really locked into the compulsions of their disease and are much less likely to be either willing or able to turn it around themselves," Dr. Yager says.

There are two main approaches to hospital programs, Dr. Mann says: traditional psychiatric treatment, and the newer 12-step treatment program fashioned after Alcoholics Anonymous, where patients are taught to face their problem and control it, step by step. "It requires you to sign on to the 12-step philosophy, which is based on acknowledging and relying on a higher power outside yourself," says Dr. Mann.

ENDOMETRIOSIS

As if those monthly cramps weren't enough, now your period has been punctuated with new pain: Maybe your lower back aches more than an overaggressive bellboy's or you feel pain during bowel movements or sex.

Your doctor may tell you it's endometriosis, a condition that occurs when the tissue that lines the uterus becomes implanted on other pelvic organs—usually on the ovaries, the fallopian tubes or the ligaments that support your uterus. It may affect the bowel, bladder or ureters as well. This misguided tissue imitates the menstrual cycle, leaving a discharge that can't exit the body and causing inflammation and scarring. It can also cause infertility in a small percentage of women.

Pregnancy and breastfeeding can end symptoms of endometriosis, but here are some easier and faster ways to get relief.

Get into workouts. While a rigorous workout may be the last thing on your mind when pain strikes, plenty of exercise is often recommended. Research shows that women who exercise regularly have less endometriosis pain and easier periods in general.

"Exercise decreases estrogen production—and estrogen makes the disease worse," explains Owen Montgomery, M.D., an obstetrics and gynecology specialist at Thomas Jefferson University Hospital and Jefferson Medical College of Thomas Jefferson University, both in Philadelphia. His recommendation: a *vigorous* workout three to six times a week for at least 30 minutes each time.

Eat for a stronger immune system. Just as diet influences the severity of other diseases, it may have a role in causing endometriosis pain. "There is data suggesting an association of autoimmune disease with both the risk of developing endometriosis and the extent or severity of endometriosis," says Dan Martin, M.D., clinical associate professor of obstetrics and gynecology at the University of Tennessee and a reproductive surgeon at Baptist Memorial Hospital, both in Memphis. To build a stronger immune system, eat plenty of fresh fruits and vegetables that are rich in vitamins. Vitamin C is especially important, so fill up your plate with vegetables and fruits such as broccoli, red bell peppers, oranges, strawberries and cantaloupe—all high in vitamin C.

Don't forget fish. Rich in omega-3 fatty acids, fish such as mackerel, herring and sardines are also helpful, because they suppress prostaglandin production, suggests gynecology and fertility specialist Camran Nezhat, M.D., director of the Fertility and Endoscopy Center and Center for Special Pelvic Surgery in Atlanta. Prostaglandin is a hormone in the uterine lining that causes cramping.

Try hands-on healing. Acupressure relieves pain in some women, says Susan Anderson, an endometriosis sufferer who is a member of the national board of the Endometriosis Association, a self-help group based in Milwaukee. When pain begins, press the area on the inside of your leg about two inches above your ankle bone. To locate that spot, press with your thumb until you locate an area that feels tender. Another spot where pressure can ease pain is the web of your hand, at the base where the bones of your thumb and index finger meet. "If it doesn't hurt when you press, then it's not the right spot. Know that it will hurt, but you need to keep pressing, and you should feel relief in the pelvic area," says Anderson.

Keep a calendar of symptoms. If you know when endometriosis pain is likely to occur each month, you can plan around it. Dr. Montgomery recommends keeping a chart of your symptoms for a few months until you see a pattern.

"Charting helps you get control of your disease, so you can plan your life better," he says. "For instance, if you know that you always have severe pain on the 22nd day of your cycle, you can avoid planning important events for that day. You can also plan your pain relief medications prior to that day, so you won't wake up on the 22nd day with severe pain."

Switch off caffeine and nicotine. Caffeine found in coffee, tea, chocolate and cola has been found to aggravate symptoms, says Dr. Nezhat. And while there's no scientific proof, most experts suspect that smoking aggravates endometriosis symptoms and pain. If you smoke and drink coffee or tea, consider giving them up—at least during your period.

Block the prostaglandin. One of the reasons for cramping, especially at the time of your period, is that your body produces too much prostaglandin, a hormone in the uterine lining. It overstimulates your uterine muscles, forcing them to work overtime. And, like any muscle that works too hard, they cramp. Aspirin, an anti-inflammatory drug, may relieve cramps, but the best over-the-counter pain relievers are anti-prostaglandins such as Advil, Medipren or Nuprin. Take two tablets at a time, says Dr. Nezhat.

Heat yourself up. Taking ibuprofen (Advil) is probably the easiest thing to do, but many women find a heating pad and warm beverages bring relief from abdominal pain and cramping, says Mary Sinn, R.N., nurse manager of the Medical Surgical Department and former coordinator of the WomanCare Unit at Gnaden Huetten Hospital in Lehighton, Pennsylvania.

Or cool yourself down. If heat doesn't help you beat endometriosis, you may be among those women who get more relief from an ice pack placed on your lower abdominal area, adds Sinn.

FIBROCYSTIC BREASTS

During a woman's childbearing years, it's very likely that she will develop numerous harmless lumps in one or both breasts, a condition often called fibrocystic breasts, one form of benign breast disease. The lumps typically occur in clumps, so your breasts may feel as though there are bunches of peas (or grapes) just under the surface. Sometimes it can feel like one lump.

Doctors aren't sure what causes fibrocystic breasts, but the condition probably is related to fluctuations of the hormones estrogen and progesterone during a woman's menstrual cycle. In fact, when women stop menstruating after menopause, the lumps may disappear. Fibrocystic lumps are not dangerous, but they can become quite sore as your period approaches. They may hurt at other times as well.

"The large majority of women have some pain in their breasts before their period starts," says David P. Rose, M.D., Ph.D., chief of the Division of Nutrition and Endocrinology at the Naylor Dana Institute in Valhalla, New York. "It is such a common finding that it really can't be considered a disease."

To understand just how common fibrocystic breasts are, consider this: If ten of your friends had a careful breast exam, at least five might have *detectable* fibrocystic lumps. The others might have fibrocystic lumps too small to be felt. If a doctor proceeded to inspect their breast tissue under a microscope, he might very well find fibrocystic changes in at least nine cases.

This doesn't mean you can ignore any new lump that appears in your breast, Dr. Rose stresses. Statistically, it probably isn't cancer, but you need a medical examination and occasionally a biopsy to be sure.

A diagnosis of fibrocystic breasts doesn't necessarily mean you have to live with pain each month. Here's what doctors recommend you do.

Lumps That Aren't Cancer

Cancer of the breast kills more women than any other kind of cancer except lung cancer. That's why it's so important that you call your doctor *immediately* if you discover a lump. Fortunately, most lumps aren't cancer, even though you fear that yours is. In most cases, what you're feeling beneath the surface is benign breast disease—harmless lumps, says David P. Rose, M.D., Ph.D., of the Naylor Dana Institute in Valhalla, New York. Sometimes your doctor will only perform an examination in making a diagnosis. Occasionally, a biopsy or mammogram will also be recommended. There are many types of noncancerous breast lumps.

- Cysts. These fluid-filled sacs usually get larger before your period, shrink when it's over and disappear after menopause. Some cysts are too small to feel; others can be a few inches across. If your doctor decides to withdraw fluid from a cyst, it will often collapse like a water balloon with the water let out.
- Fibroadenomas. These round, rubbery lumps freely slide around inside the breast. Common in younger women, they often get larger during pregnancy and when you breast-feed. Even your doctor can mistake a fibroadenoma for a more dangerous tumor. Your doctor may remove it just to be on the safe side.
- Lipomas. These small, soft, painless, slow-growing lumps are often found in older women. Consisting of fatty tissue, they slide freely in the breast. Lipomas often are removed or biopsied to check for cancer.
- Intraductal papillomas. Relatively rare, these small growths can appear in the lining of the ducts near the nipple and will occasionally cause bleeding. Such bleeding should never be ignored. As with lipomas and fibroadenomas, your doctor may remove them just to be sure they're harmless.

Cut the caffeine. Some researchers suggest that caffeine not only gives you a morning jump-start but also can stimulate changes in your breasts. In one study, for example, 113 women with fibrocystic breasts were asked to forgo their morning brew. After one year, nearly two out of three said they had less breast pain than before.

However, quite a few doctors aren't convinced that coffee makes a difference, Dr. Rose says. "The large studies would suggest that there isn't a relationship between caffeine and fibrocystic breasts. Yet we all know of patients who swear they had trouble with breast pain until they cut out caffeine—which to me is a good reason for trying it," he says.

Forgo the fat, fill up on fiber. Women with high levels of the hormone estrogen may be at risk for developing fibrocystic breasts, Dr. Rose says. "You can reduce the circulating levels of estrogen by going on a low-fat, high-fiber diet," he says.

Try vitamin E for aches. Several studies have suggested that daily doses of vitamin E may reduce both the pain of fibrocystic breasts and the size of the lumps. As with caffeine, however, some doctors aren't convinced that it really works. If you decide to give vitamin E a try, ask your doctor to recommend a safe dose— 400 international units (IUs) a day or less. In large doses, vitamin E can be toxic.

Break in a new bra. Exercise bras, sometimes called jogging bras, can relieve tenderness by giving your breasts extra support during the last days of your menstrual cycle.

Try some OTC relief. On particularly bad days, over-the-counter painkillers such as aspirin and ibuprofen can help.

FIBROIDS

When Ellen was 35 and had recently moved to Sarasota, Florida, she noticed that her periods were gradually getting longer. She was bleeding more, too, sometimes soaking through a dozen tampons a day. "That was the summer I took up roots and started my new job, so I figured I was just stressed out," remembers Ellen, now 40. By the fall, however, she was feeling much calmer—yet the bleeding was still heavy. Finally she made an appointment to see her gynecologist.

"Is something . . . wrong?" Ellen nervously asked.

"What you have are fibroids," her doctor replied. "But don't worry. It's probably not a serious problem."

Also called leomyomas, uterine fibroids are common tumors that affect as many as one in four women during their reproductive years, says Julia V. Johnson, M.D., an assistant professor of obstetrics and gynecology at the University of Vermont in Burlington. Composed of normal uterine musculature and fueled by the hormone estrogen, fibroids can be as small as a seed or as large as a melon. They grow inside or outside the uterus, sometimes attached by stalks, like mushrooms.

For many women, fibroids never cause symptoms. In fact, smaller fibroids are often discovered "accidentally" during routine pelvic examinations. But those that grow to look more like melons than seeds can cause a host of problems. For example, some women notice they're getting bigger around the middle, even though they're not gaining weight. Some others have low backaches. "Probably the most common symptoms are pelvic pain and heavy bleeding during the period," Dr. Johnson says.

Fibroids may also worsen during pregnancy. In some circumstances, they can actually obstruct labor. Large fibroids sometimes degenerate or cause acute pain during pregnancy. Conversely, fibroids inside the uterus that distort the uterine cavity (called subserousal fibroids) may occasionally prohibit pregnancy from occurring.

If the word *tumor* makes you think of cancer—*relax*. Fewer than 1 in 200 uterine fibroids ever becomes cancerous. "In fact, it's unknown if fibroids actually turn into cancer or if there just happen to be cancers that coexist with the fibroids," says Dr. Johnson.

Be aware of the fat factor. Since fibroids depend on estrogen for their development and growth, in theory it may be possible to control them merely by watching your weight, says Richard J. Worley, M.D., an associate clinical professor of obstetrics and gynecology at the University of Colorado Health Science Center in Denver. This is because estrogen is produced not only by the ovaries but by fat tissue as well. "Obese women produce more estrogen in fat tissue than do slender women," explains Dr. Worley.

When researchers from Harvard Medical School studied the hospital records of 144 women who had surgery for fibroids, they found that 51 percent were obese. The researchers defined obese as 20 percent or more above ideal body weight. By contrast, only 25 percent of all American women are overweight.

Although doctors aren't yet certain that obesity stimulates fibroid growth, it does appear to be one risk factor that women can control, Dr. Worley says. "Given a genetic predisposition to fibroids, the ability of obesity to add to the estrogen in the system certainly could be a factor."

Options to consider. Many women with fibroids will never need treatment. "If the fibroids are relatively small and they're not producing any symptoms, then you may want to just follow them and see if they get worse," says Dr. Johnson. But if they are causing problems, "then removing them is going to be the way to go."

Doctors in the past typically treated symptomatic fibroids by removing the entire uterus, an operation called hysterectomy. While hysterectomy still is the most definitive treatment for fibroids—once the uterus is removed, fibroids can't come back—it obviously won't do for women who still want to have children, Dr. Worley says.

Instead of hysterectomy, doctors often recommend myomectomy, an operation that removes the fibroids while leaving the uterus intact. This is often done by making an abdominal incision to expose the uterus, then opening the uterus to remove the fibroids. This procedure takes about 90 minutes, and women can usually return home within a few days, Dr. Worley says. A relatively new technique for removing fibroids from inside the uterus is even simpler. A surgeon can remove the fibroid by inserting a telescope-like instrument (hysteroscope) through the cervix and into the uterus. Women often return home the same day. "It's quite a straightforward and predictable operation," explains Dr. Worley.

For all of the benefits, there is one problem with either kind of technique: The fibroids often come back. "The risk of recurrence can be as high as 30 percent," Dr. Johnson says. For a young woman, this could mean having several operations before reaching menopause. But for older women already approaching menopause, the one operation will probably be all they need. (After menopause, estrogen-starved fibroids usually shrink on their own.)

HANGNAIL

A tiny sliver of skin splits off from your fingernail. And there it hangs, a little skin-thick piece of pain just waiting to happen. The trouble is, when a hangnail catches on something, this most minor of injuries can cause major-league pain.

The best way to avoid hangnails (which have nothing to do with the nails themselves) is by keeping your hands well moisturized. The splits usually occur when the skin around the nails dries up and dies; nail biting is another common cause. Here are some of the best ways to cure them.

Soak before clipping. "A lot of people make the mistake of clipping a hangnail when it's still hard and dry and end up ripping the skin more," says Trisha Webster, a hand model with the Wilhelmina Modeling Agency in New York City whose livelihood depends on perfectly groomed hands. "So before you clip a hangnail, soak it in a little water—or a water-and-oil solution—to soften it." To make the solution, just add two capfuls of mild bath oil or two tablespoons of olive oil to a bowl of warm water.

Clip and cover. "The best thing to do with a hangnail is clip the little piece of skin with a pair of nail scissors—but be sure to wipe the scissors with rubbing alcohol before using them," advises Karen E. Burke, M.D., Ph.D., a dermatologist and dermatologic surgeon in New York City. "Then put on an antibacterial ointment to prevent infection, and cover your finger with a bandage."

Go for soaks. Soaking your nails in a mixture of oil and water on a regular basis is a good way to make sure you don't get future hangnails. Regular water-and-oil soaks replenish lost moisture. "I tell my patients to mix four capfuls of bath oil such as Alpha Keri with one pint of warm water and to soak their fingertips in it for maybe 10 or 15 minutes," says Rodney Basler, M.D., a dermatologist and assistant professor of internal medicine at the University of Nebraska Medical Center in Omaha.

Wrap it up. It's a good idea to bandage your finger after removing a hangnail, but if the bandage falls off (because of the moisturizing soak), wrap your finger in a piece of plastic wrap and secure the wrap with some tape, advises Dr. Basler. "The plastic will keep the moisture in overnight. Just be sure to remove the plastic in the morning, because you don't want to keep it on too long."

Take Mom's advice. "I advise the same thing your mother told you: Don't bite hangnails," says Dr. Basler. "If you bite them, you end up with fairly deep cuts around your fingers. And those can get infected."

Cuticle cautions. Because hangnails often form around the cuticle, many people try to avoid them by using cuticle-removing solutions. That's not a good idea, says Diana Bihova, M.D., a dermatologist and clinical instructor of dermatology at the New York University Medical Center in New York City.

"Many of these products, which are designed to tame excess or ragged cuticles, contain sodium hydroxide," she explains. "This caustic chemical can destroy skin tissue, so products containing it can cause irritation if left on too long. Use such products sparingly and always follow package instructions carefully. It's the cuticle, after all, that provides the vital function of protecting your nails from harmful bacteria and fungi.

"Hangnails sound very innocent," she warns, "but if they get infected, they can lead to serious inflammation of the cuticles and other tissues surrounding the nails."

HOT FLASHES

As a woman reaches menopause—usually around age 50—hormone levels fall rapidly as the ovaries halt production of the hormone estrogen. Sensing this, the body's internal thermostat tends to react quite strongly. Blood vessels on the skin's surface open up like a radiator, enveloping you in intense heat and flushing your face. About 80 percent of all women experience these hot flashes as they go through menopause.

Your doctor may prescribe estrogen tablets if your hot flashes are severe. But many women find they can deal with milder symptoms with home treatments.

Track those flashes. Hot flashes may occur more predictably and less randomly than you think, studies show. To prove it, take note of the date, time, intensity and duration of the hot flash, suggests Linda Gannon, Ph.D., professor of psychology at Southern Illinois University at Carbondale. Also record the circumstances preceding it—what you ate or drank, how you felt emotionally.

"Some women find that hot flashes worsen when they drink alcohol or coffee, smoke cigarettes or encounter stressful situations that elicit strong emotions," says Dr. Gannon. Your hot flash diary can show you what triggers you need to avoid to keep cool.

Lower the temp. Keeping cool is important for menopausal women, since many of the precipitating factors in hot flashes are related to heat, says Sadja Greenwood, M.D., assistant clinical professor of gynecology at the University of California, San Francisco, Medical Center. She suggests sipping cool drinks and wearing natural fabrics that "breathe." And one Columbia University study showed that menopausal women had fewer and milder hot flashes in cool rooms than in hot rooms. So turn on the fan or the air conditioner to keep the temperature down. And when you're going out, carry a fold-up fan with you, Dr. Greenwood advises.

Keep a cool head—meditate. Some brain research has shown that hot flashes are stimulated by a brain chemical (neurotransmitter) known as norepinephrine, which influences the temperature-regulating center in the brain, says Dr. Greenwood. "This may explain why daily stress reduction practices such as meditation, deep breathing and yoga, which result in lower levels of norepinephrine, help some women reduce their hot flashes," she says.

In one study, menopausal women with frequent hot flashes were trained to slowly breathe in and out six to eight times for two minutes. These women had fewer hot flashes than women trained to use either muscle relaxation or biofeedback.

Douse it with vitamin E. "This nutrient often does a commendable job of relieving the severity and frequency of flashes. Lots of my patients have good luck with it," says Lila E. Nachtigall, M.D., associate professor of obstetrics and gynecology at New York University School of Medicine in New York City. She recommends starting with 400 international units twice a day (a total of 800 international units).

But check with your physician before beginning vitamin E supplementation. While the vitamin is generally considered safe, it can have a blood-thinning effect. Meanwhile, try to include more vitamin E–rich foods in your diet: wheat germ, wheat germ oil, safflower oil, whole-grain breads and cereals, peanuts, walnuts, filberts and almonds.

Sip some sarsaparilla. For centuries, herbalists have used special "women's herbs" that have a weak regulating effect on estrogen and may help control hot flashes, according to Susan Lark, M.D., medical director of the PMS and Menopause Self-Help Center in Los Altos, California. The herbs include sarsaparilla, dong quoi, black cohosh, false unicorn root, fennel and anise.

These herbs are available combined in ready-made formulas, or they can be used alone, says Dr. Lark. To make a tea, empty one herb capsule into a cup of boiling water and let it steep for a few minutes. Don't drink more than two cups of herbal tea (along with meals) daily. Discontinue the herbs if you notice nausea or other symptoms, says Dr. Lark. And talk to your doctor before taking these herbs if you're at risk for cancer or other conditions that rule out estrogen replacement therapy.

Get up and go. In one Swedish study, severe hot flashes and night sweats were only half as common among physically active postmenopausal women as among bench warmers. "Possibly, exercise elevates the level of endorphins, the feel-good hormones that drop when there is an estrogen deficiency," says Timothy Yeko, M.D., assistant professor in the Department of Obstetrics and Gynecology, Division of Reproductive Endocrinology, at the University of South Florida in Tampa. The endorphins affect the thermoregulatory center—your thermostat, says Dr. Yeko. Regular physical activity may increase endorphin activity and therefore diminish the frequency of hot flashes.

Don't aim to be a skinny-mini. "Estrogen is actually manufactured in body fat from other hormones after menopause," says Dr. Greenwood. "A very thin woman will have less natural estrogen in her system, which may give her more problems with hot flashes."

INHIBITED SEXUAL DESIRE

You've lost that loving feeling. It's gone, gone, gone, and nothing you do seems to get it back.

Well, there's no reason to believe it's gone forever. Usually the lack of sexual interest is only temporary. In fact, it's a normal reaction to stress, illness, hormonal swings or emotional upset.

But what happens when there's not even a flicker of renewed interest? That is a condition psychologists call inhibited sexual desire.

"People with inhibited sexual desire lack the desire to have sex, even though they have opportunities to do so," explains Shirley Zussman, Ed.D., a marital therapist in New York City. "In some instances, they completely lose interest in sex." Or their interest in sex may change dramatically over a period of months.

Of course, not everyone considers a low libido a problem. But some do, and more than a fair number of people with a low sex drive have spouses who consider it a big problem, says Peter A. Wish, Ph.D., director of the New England Institute of Family Relations in Framingham, Massachusetts.

If you're among them, here are some tips that may help you rekindle your flame and help you and your mate adjust to each other's differing appetites.

Exercise your options. Studies have shown that exercisers tend to enjoy sex more than nonexercisers. Regular, strenuous exercise may be a potent aphrodisiac, helping to boost your love life. "Exercise may also help people feel better about themselves and the way they look," says David McWhirter, M.D., professor of psychiatry at the University of California in San Diego.

Make a date. "No time for sex is a frequent complaint, so make it a priority by making time," Dr. Zussman suggests. Be playful and creative, and start "dating" again. Go to a drive-in movie on a hot, humid night. Watch the sun set. Snuggle up together under the blankets with a good book. Hide from the kids the same way you used to hide from your parents when you were teenagers. Leave notes, send cards, give gifts, bring home flowers just for the joy of it.

Catch some rays. There's no doubt that a day of sunshine can lift your spirits. But did you know that exposure to the sun may be sexually stimulating, too?

Researchers at the University of Texas Health Science Center at San Antonio found that a person who gets a lot of sunlight has a stronger sex drive. Not only that, sunlight increases ovulation in women and sperm production in men. "Get out in the sunlight for a half-hour or so at midday during the winter months," suggests Russell J. Reiter, M.D., Ph.D., professor of neuroendocrinology at the health science center.

And keep your living space bright by opening the curtains to let in natural sunlight and using high-wattage bulbs.

Try to work it out. "Many sex drive problems are really intimacy problems," Dr. Wish says. "There might be anger, unresolved conflicts or any one of a number of things that are incomplete." He emphasizes that it's important to talk about these things in a supportive way.

Accentuate the positive. Pick a place far removed from the bedroom to have a discussion, suggests Dr. Zussman. "Start out not in an angry way but by affirming what's positive about the relationship," she suggests. "You may want to begin with 'We have so many good things between us, and this seems to be one area that just isn't working right.' People are very vulnerable about their lack of sexual interest, and it does no good to attack them for it."

Discover the whole body. Couples who concentrate on just reaching orgasm deprive themselves of prolonged pleasures. Do more touching, hugging and hand-holding, Dr. Zussman suggests.

A SEX RX

I f you find you can't even broach the subject with your mate, or if sex isn't the only thing you are no longer able to enjoy, you may benefit from discussing your problem with a professional. You can ask your family doctor, a gynecologist or a urologist for a referral.

Doctors recommend that you address both the psychological and physical aspects of inhibited sexual desire. Individual therapy or a medical checkup might be advised before marital therapy. Inhibited sexual desire can be a symptom of depression. It can also be due to low hormone levels, which are best diagnosed and treated by an endocrinologist, who specializes in the body's internal secretion system.

Read the fine print on drugs you're taking. Some drugs crimp not only sexual performance but sexual desire as well. Common lust busters: anti-anxiety and sleep-inducing drugs and some blood pressure medications. Ask your doctor about side effects. He may be able to substitute a drug with fewer desire-dampening effects.

IRON-DEFICIENCY ANEMIA

Are you fatigued? Short of breath? Chilly?

If so, worries about your health and state of mind have probably led you to the doctor's door already. And if you're a woman in your thirties or forties, there's a good chance the doctor told you that you have iron-deficiency anemia. That is the kind of anemia that occurs when the iron supply, which usually carries oxygen and carbon dioxide through the body, is depleted.

Not *all* premenopausal women suffer from iron-deficiency anemia, but they are more likely to have this problem than younger women—and much more likely than men, according to M. T. Atallah, Ph.D., associate professor of nutrition at the University of Massachusetts Department of Food Science and Nutrition in Amherst.

Nutrition research has also shown that women usually need higher than usual doses of iron when they are menstruating, pregnant or lactating. But all of us tend to require more iron as we get older than we did as youngsters.

So even if you don't have full-blown iron-deficiency anemia, you may need more iron to ward off the feelings of chilliness or fatigue that people often get when the iron supply in their bodies is depleted.

Eating food that's high in iron is not the entire answer, however. You need to get iron in a form that is absorbable by the body, which means you need to be choosy about your food sources.

Some foods have a good supply of *heme* iron, which is readily absorbable. But in other foods, iron is in the *nonheme* form, which the body has trouble absorbing. Yet here's the twist: Even nonheme iron can be absorbed more readily if it's eaten with certain foods.

Hard to absorb that information? No harder than the iron itself if you heed these tips from the experts.

Eat more lean meat. "The basic answer to anemia is to eat a balanced diet while increasing the amount of meat, which is high in heme iron," says John Beard, Ph.D., professor of nutrition at Pennsylvania State University in University Park.

Make OJ part of your meals. For better absorption of the nonheme iron that's contained in plant foods such as vegetables and grains, add citrus juice to your meals. Though absorption of iron from plant sources or iron-fortified cereals is normally between 2 and 10 percent, you can almost *double* that rate if you consume a vitamin C–rich food or drink at the same time. So a glass of orange or grapefruit juice with your iron-fortified breakfast cereal means more iron for your body, according to Dr. Atallah.

Look for the iron bonuses. Iron-fortified cereals such as Cream of Wheat, raisin bran and wheat and bran flakes are excellent sources of nonheme iron, though you will need vitamin C for optimum absorption. Legumes such as soybeans are also high in nonheme iron. Carrots, potatoes, broccoli and tomatoes are other excellent plant sources of iron.

Steer clear of the iron-blocking veggies. Some vegetable sources contain a large amount of iron but also a substance called phytate, which blocks iron's ability to be absorbed. The high-phytate crowd includes butter beans, lentils, beet greens, spinach and other leafy vegetables. So if it's iron you need, don't eat these veggies with your chicken and burgers. The amount of phytate will block the heme iron absorption.

Avoid coffee or tea during meals. "It's best not to have coffee or tea with a meal if you are trying to prevent iron deficiency," says Gregory Landry, M.D., associate professor in the Department of Pediatrics at the University of Wisconsin Medical School in Madison and the head medical team physician at the university's sports clinic. These beverages contain chemicals that block iron absorption.

Be choosy with supplements. Look for an iron supplement made from ferrous gluconate instead of ferrous sulfate. It's easier on the stomach, says Dr. Landry. And avoid taking calcium supplements along with iron. "All-in-one supplements containing iron are *not* recommended," says Dr. Beard, "because the other vitamins can interfere with your body's ability to absorb iron." If you take both calcium and iron supplements, take the calcium in the morning, and take the iron supplement at night.

Take supplements with citrus sips. If you're taking an iron supplement, do your body a favor and wash it down with citrus juice, which helps the body absorb it.

Look for reduced iron. Reduced iron is often added to processed foods, such as cereals. But in spite of its negative name, it's actually a plus. "Generally, reduced iron would have *higher* availability to the body than regular iron," says Dr. Atallah.

Cook spaghetti sauce in an iron pot. When you use an iron pot for cooking, some of the iron will migrate into the food—and into your body. But not all foods have an ironclad guarantee of mining iron from the pot. The key is acidity. "If you are cooking tomato sauce, the amount of iron you'll get is high because of the acidity of the sauce," says Dr. Atallah.

MENOPAUSAL PROBLEMS

Do you have PMZ?

No, not PMS—that's premenstrual syndrome. When you say PMZ, think liberation, not liability.

PMZ stands for postmenopausal zest, a phrase coined by anthropologist Margaret Mead. And what she meant was that women should seize this stage of life and live it to the fullest. You are now unencumbered by contraception and pregnancy and that once-a-month cycle that used to slow you down. *This*, she says, is freedom.

"It's a time for exploring what it feels like to be a woman in the human sense, not just as someone who raises children," says Irene Simpson, a naturopathic practitioner in Arlington, Washington. "My friends and I are on the verge of menopause and we are finding it very empowering. We are finding personal growth at a time when women used to decline."

Menopause begins when your ovaries no longer function, when estrogen secretion slows, then stops, and monthly menstruation becomes irregular, then ceases. Normally, women reach menopause by age 51.

During the six months to three years of this cycle of your life, you may feel some of the traditional symptoms of menopause, including hot flashes and sudden chills, lowered sexual desire, vaginal dryness, emotional upset and sleeping problems. Menopause can be bittersweet. Or, it can be a time of PMZ, with an emphasis on the Zest. Here's how.

Design your own zest! Education about physiological changes and an adventurous outlook can make a big difference in handling the stresses that come with menopause, as well as the life changes (children moving out, parents moving in, for example) that many women are faced with in their late forties and early fifties, says Simpson.

Research shows that today's woman spends a third of her life postmenopausal. So consider menopause a step forward in life and make a change for the better, Simpson says. Go back to school. Find a new hobby. Change careers. Take charge of your own health. Make life an adventure.

Find support. Support groups offer reassurance that menopause is a natural cycle, says Sadja Greenwood, M.D., a family physician in San Francisco, and author of *Menopause, Naturally.* Members can offer practical coping techniques that they've discovered, as well as sisterly support for new endeavors. To find a support group, call your local women's center. To start one, place an ad in the newspaper or tack a notice on a bulletin board where women congregate, such as the YWCA.

Exercise daily. Walking, jogging, bicycling, jumping rope, dancing, swimming or any other daily exercise can relieve a lot of the symptoms of menopause, according to a study at the University of Medicine and Dentistry of New Jersey Robert Wood Johnson Medical School. Exercise can help prevent or lessen symptoms such as hot flashes and night sweats, depression and other emotional problems, as well as vaginal problems.

Improved physical fitness, of course, is the most obvious result of exercise. But exercise also improves psychological health by boosting brain concentrations of the neurotransmitters norepinephrine and serotonin, according to Gloria A. Bachmann, M.D., an associate professor of medicine in the Department of Obstetrics and Gynecology at University of Medicine and Dentistry of New Jersey Robert Wood Johnson Medical School.

She recommends aerobics and stretching exercises for flexibility, muscle strengthening and relaxation. Yoga, she reports, also aids flexibility and has an added benefit—it improves diaphragmatic breathing, which induces relaxation and reduces stress.

Lubricate your love. Vaginal dryness from a lack of estrogen decreases interest in intercourse during menopause, says Marilyn Poland, R.N., Ph.D., an associate professor of gynecology and obstetrics at Wayne State University School of Medicine. A water-soluable lubricant, such as Lubifax or K-Y jelly, vegetable oils and unscented cream or oil are all good choices for lubrication, says Dr. Greenwood.

Or break open a couple of capsules of vitamin E and massage them on as a lubricant, says Simpson.

Make talk. Talk to your partner, advises Simpson. Some libido boosting comes with heart-to-heart talks about needs and feelings.

Take high adventure to the bedroom. Couples may want to try new positions in intercourse to find the most comfortable, says Dr. Greenwood. Touching can be especially important at this time. She suggests more hugs and mutual massages for closeness and sensual pleasure.

Do the Kegel. You can strengthen your anal, vaginal and urinary muscles with a special exercise called a Kegel, says Simpson. Stronger muscles can help you relax and use these muscles with less pain and more pleasure during intercourse. They are also good for preventing urinary incontinence, a problem for some menopausal women. Here's how to do it.

Imagine you want to stop urine in midstream. Squeeze the muscles in your vaginal area firmly. Hold to the count of three, then relax. Practice with a rapid alternation between tightening and letting go. You can practice this exercise anywhere, anytime.

MENSTRUAL CRAMPS

People who think "What's the big deal?" when it comes to menstrual cramps obviously haven't had to deal with a full-blown case of these gut-grabbing spasms.

The pain can feel like an abdominal charley horse, and worse yet, this time of month may bring on diarrhea and nausea. Admittedly, menstrual cramps do tend to ease off within a day or two, but who wants 48 hours of misery if it can possibly be avoided?

When pain is that intense, doctors recommend a checkup to make sure your menstrual cramps aren't being caused by something that may require medical treatment, such as endometriosis or a pelvic infection, says Penny Wise Budoff, M.D., director of the Women's Health Services affiliated with the North Shore University Hospital in Bethpage, New York, and author of *No More Menstrual Cramps and Other Good News.*

But once you've ruled out other causes, here are some techniques to maximize comfort and minimize monthly pain.

Mind your minerals. The minerals calcium, potassium and magnesium can also play a part in relief, says Susan Lark, M.D., director of the PMS Self-Help Center in Los Altos, California. She says she has found that women taking calcium suffer less pain from cramps than those who do not. Magnesium is important, she notes, because it helps your body absorb calcium more efficiently. She suggests increasing calcium and magnesium intake before and during your period.

Say yes to drugs. Nonsteroidal anti-inflammatory drugs such as ibuprofen (Advil) work best to relieve menstrual cramps, and they may also take the edge off the breast pain and sometimes the diarrhea that go along with cramps. That's because these drugs inhibit the formation of prostaglandins, chemicals that cause muscle cramps and pain.

"The trick to easing your pain is to take medication at the very onset of pain or discomfort and repeat every six hours until the pain subsides," says Andrea Rapkin, M.D., associate professor of obstetrics and gynecology at the University of California, Los Angeles, School of Medicine. "Don't save the medication for times of severe pain."

Walk it off. Exercise is a muscle tension reducer and a mood elevator. And it may reduce menstrual cramps by improving circulation in the pelvic organs, experts say. "If you're walking, strike a relaxed pose that lets you swing your hips and arms freely and lets you breathe rhythmically," suggests Robert Thayer, Ph.D., professor of psychology at California State University, Long Beach. If your normally brisk pace wears you out during this time, do yourself a favor and slow down, he adds.

Seek heat. A warm bath or a heating pad on your belly or the small of your back can relax muscle spasms and ease cramping pain, according to doctors. When you're walking outdoors in cold weather, wear a warm jacket that reaches below your hips. That will help keep pelvic muscles warm and relaxed.

Strike a diamond pose. Yoga can provide exceptional pain relief for menstrual cramps, says Patricia Hammond, a yoga instructor and director of the Sarasota Center of the American Yoga Association in Sarasota, Florida. "We recommend a light routine that stretches and limbers the hips and other joints but doesn't vigorously compress or stretch the abdomen," she says.

Try this pose: Sit on the floor with your back erect. Bend your knees, keeping them as close to the floor as possible. Bring your feet together, sole to sole, making a diamond shape with your legs. Keeping your back straight, breathe in, then slowly bend forward as you exhale. Breathe in and straighten. Bend forward again as you exhale. Repeat several times—feel yourself sink lower with each exhalation.

Curl up in a ball. Here's another yoga pose that's a sure-bet cramp reliever. Kneel, then sit back so that your buttocks rest on your heels and bend forward to rest your chest on your thighs.

Place your forehead on the floor, with your arms stretched in back of you so that your hands are by your feet. If your head doesn't touch the floor comfortably, rest it on your folded arms. Breathe normally, and as you exhale, imagine your whole body becoming more limp and relaxed.

If this pose is uncomfortable, you can do a modified version of this pose in a chair, Hammond says. "Sit way back in the chair, with your feet flat on the floor, and lean forward, wrapping your arms around your knees or lower legs." If this pose is uncomfortable, simply rest your arms on top of your knees.

Stretch your iliopsoas. No, it's not some sort of strange tropical vine. The iliopsoas are three muscles (major, minor and iliacus) on both sides of your pelvis, stretching from your lower spine to your femur—the upper thigh bone. Tight 'psoas have been implicated in a variety of pelvic organ disorders, including painful menstrual cramps, says Robert King, co-director of the Chicago School of Massage Therapy and a nationally certified massage therapist. To make it easier to stand up straight and to open the area between your ribs and hipbone, you need to stretch these muscles, King says. Here's how.

In a partial side lunge, spread your feet apart and turn your body over the trailing leg, partially bending the knees, then lunge to the other side and repeat. This stretches the musculature of the pelvic area and the 'psoas.

Drink some herbal tea. Gingerroot tea can help relieve menstrual cramps. To make it, slice a handful of gingerroot and simmer it in water for 15 minutes.

MIGRAINES

Referring to a migraine as a headache is like saying the Grand Canyon is a large hole. While a run-of-the-mill headache can make your head spin, migraines can make you feel like Linda Blair in *The Exorcist.* Besides intense head pain, there's often nausea and vomiting as well.

The onset of a migraine is not like the creeping-in head pain of the "classic" tension headache. About 20 minutes before the war between your ears, a migraine can cause flashes of light, blind spots, dazzling zigzag lines, dizziness and numbness on one side of the body. You may feel thirsty or crave sweets, feel elated and energetic or drowsy and depressed. There's also hypersentivity to light and sound.

Heredity plays a role, and women are twice as likely as men to suffer migraines. These mega-headaches usually start around puberty and tend to dwindle after age 45. (But for some reason, they rarely occur during pregnancy.) Although the exact cause of migraines is unknown, evidence suggests that these one-sided headaches (they don't affect the *entire* skull) have something to do with the blood vessels in your head. Triggers also include certain foods, stress, light and even perfumes or other odors.

Your doctor may prescribe ergotamine for these hard-to-handle headaches, but that drug can produce distressing symptoms of its own. Luckily, the experts say, there are other ways to control migraines.

Sleep it off. "Generally, the best treatment for a migraine is to sleep," says Glen Solomon, M.D., a headache specialist at the Cleveland Clinic Foundation in Cleveland and associate professor of medicine at Ohio State University in Columbus. "Relief comes from falling asleep—even if it's for a short time." Dr. Solomon warns, however, that napping can trigger other types of headaches. So if you're susceptible to other headaches besides migraines, the best policy is to get on a regular sleeping schedule rather than take catnaps.

Say no to NutraSweet. The popular artificial sweetener isn't so sweet to migraineurs: Aspartame (sold commercially as NutraSweet) can trigger migraines or make them worse. "Various studies have implicated NutraSweet but *not* other artificial sweeteners," says Fred Sheftell, M.D., director of the New England Center for Headache in Stamford, Connecticut, and coauthor of *Headache Relief*. "There's no question, medically, that many people prone to migraines or headaches will do better if they eliminate NutraSweet."

Take time to relax—literally. "Most migraines occur on weekends or while people are on vacation, and I think it may have to do with a *reduction* of stress," says Dr. Solomon. "When the body's stressed, it produces adrenaline—and adrenaline protects blood vessels against migraines. When you relax and don't have this adrenaline protection, you're more prone to an attack. You need to ease into relaxation, make it more of a gradual transition than just going full blast until 5:00 P.M. Friday and then suddenly stopping everything. I suggest practicing some sort of relaxation technique to slowly unwind—exercise, listening to music, whatever helps you relax—rather than just leaving work Friday afternoon and hitting the bar."

Munch on magnesium. Research by K. Michael Welch, M.D., a neurologist at Henry Ford Health Sciences Center in Detroit, suggests that most migraine sufferers may have a shortage of magnesium in their brains. "Magnesium is a muscle relaxer, and it can help those with migraines," says Allan Magaziner, D.O., a Cherry Hill, New Jersey, family practitioner who specializes in nutritional therapy and preventive medicine. Good sources of this mineral include dark green, leafy vegetables, fruits and nuts.

Watch what you eat. About 10 to 15 percent of people plagued by migraines are food-sensitive, which means that consuming some foods or drinks can trigger a severe migraine, says Dr. Solomon. "There are certain foods that we know are triggers—chocolate, red wine and other items containing the amino

FOODS THAT BRING PAIN

C ertain foods are known to trigger migraines in some people. Leading culprits include:

- Alcohol (especially red and fortified wines).
- Foods containing tyramine (an amino acid)—chocolate, aged cheeses, organ meats, vinegar, catsup, salad dressings, sour cream, yogurt and yeast extracts.
- Foods containing MSG (monosodium glutamate).
- Other offenders—citrus fruits, onions, dairy products, pickled herring, deli meats, hot dogs, lima/fava beans and seafood.

acid tyramine. Also, foods cooked with MSG [monosodium glutamate] can trigger attacks. I tell my patients to eat what they want but to note if they get headaches after eating certain foods. If they do, stay away from those foods."

Take an aspirin every other day. A landmark Physician's Health Study in 1989 found that aspirin reduced the risk of heart attack. Less publicized was the finding that aspirin is also very beneficial for alleviating migraines. In the 22,000-person study, migraine-prone participants who took a 325-milligram aspirin tablet every other day cut their attacks by 20 percent. "Even a *daily* dose of aspirin seems to help prevent migraines," says Seymour Diamond, M.D., executive director of the National Headache Foundation and director of the Diamond Headache Clinic in Chicago. Be sure, however, to check with your doctor before you start an aspirin-a-day program.

Try feverfew. Fevers are fewer after taking this white-flowered plant, and so are migraine headaches. Research conducted at University Hospital in Nottingham, England, has shown that people who take feverfew get fewer and less intense migraines. You can grow feverfew, a common herb, or check your local health food store for supplements or powders. *Note:* Don't take feverfew if you're pregnant. And if you experience swollen lips, dulled taste buds or a sore mouth and tongue after trying the herb, be sure to stop taking it.

Ice your head. You have a 50-50 chance of getting some pain relief *within three minutes* of applying a soft, cold ice pack wrapped in a towel to your head, says Lawrence Robbins, M.D., assistant professor of neurology at Rush Medical College and the University of Illinois College of Medicine, both in Chicago, who also has his own headache clinic in Northbrook, Illinois. That's because ice constricts blood vessels, returning them back to normal size.

Be aerobically inclined. Doctors have long known that exercise is a great way to reduce the stress that often triggers migraines in some people. But now there's research suggesting that cardiovascular fitness may also help lessen migraines—no matter what the cause. Research psychologists at Carleton University in Ottawa, Ontario, report that the severity of migraines decreases as cardiovascular fitness increases. "Regular exercise is a great idea for anyone who has migraines," agrees Dr. Diamond. But he warns: Exercise *during* an attack can make it worse.

Relax—as often as possible. Whether you just "imagine" yourself on a beach or actually go to one, practicing a *regular* activity that helps you unwind, relax and manage stress is *essential* for preventing migraines, say *all* our experts. Try to find some time every day for activities such as listening to music, reading or practicing yoga.

Don't pop the Pill. If you're a migraine-prone woman who takes birth control pills, you might want to consider discontinuing them. One in three women with migraines has increased attacks when they take oral contraceptives.

MORNING SICKNESS

You had planned to be a radiant madonna, one of those pregnant women who grow more beautiful with each passing month. Morning sickness just wasn't in the game plan.

Yvonne Thornton, M.D., remembers. An assistant professor of obstetrics and gynecology at Cornell University Medical College in New York City and mother of two, she used to make light of her patients' complaints—until she knew better. "What's a little nausea, I thought. And then I became pregnant. I was camped out by the toilet every 5 minutes!"

Of course, your experience with morning sickness is probably a lot different from Dr. Thornton's. Or from anybody else's, for that matter. That's because morning sickness is different from person to person. In fact, you may not even get it in the morning. It can hit at any time during the day. Maybe you'll feel worse in the evening, after a long day at work. Maybe certain smells will trigger it.

Typically, morning sickness begins around week 6 of pregnancy, about the same time that the placenta begins serious production of human chorionic gonadotropin (HCG), a special pregnancy hormone. In most women, symptoms peak during week 8 or 9 and wane after week 13.

The good news is that morning sickness seems to be a sign that the pregnancy is going well. A National Institute of Child Health and Human Development study of 9,098 pregnant women found that women who vomited during their first trimester were less likely to miscarry or deliver prematurely.

That cheers you some. But what can you do to get through it? Here's what our experts advise.

Start your day with saltines. "The best thing is to eat some dry crackers or biscuits first thing in the morning," says John Willems, M.D., associate clinical professor of obstetrics and gynecology at the University of California, San Diego, and a researcher at the Scripps Clinic and Research Foundation in La Jolla. "You'll actually feel better if you have something in your stomach—and the best thing is some sort of dry carbohydrate." Other good foods to choose, besides crackers, include a plain, un-buttered bagel, a piece of matzo or dry toast.

Eat a little a lot. If you're prone to morning sickness, you can lessen its impact by eating five or six "small" meals a day rather than a traditional breakfast, lunch and dinner, says Jack Galloway, M.D., clinical professor of obstetrics and gynecology at the University of Southern California School of Medicine in Los Angeles.

"Morning sickness is caused by high levels of estrogen," says Dr. Galloway. "And excessive estrogen makes your stomach churn. But by constantly keeping something in your stomach, you eliminate this churning, which is caused by increased stomach acids." Eating a big meal may immediately soothe your stomach, but the churning returns several hours later when food leaves the stomach for the intestines.

Go nuts over almonds. They are high in B vitamins and contain fat and protein—what you and your baby need right now. And they help fulfill the requirement of small meals, says Deborah Gowen, a certified nurse-midwife with the Harvard Community Health Plan in Wellesley, Massachusetts.

Walk away from your problems. Stress makes morning sickness worse, which is one reason why so many working women suffer from morning sickness. "The boss is yelling at them, people calling in are yelling and when they go home, their husbands yell at them, too," says Dr. Galloway. "You can bet they'll feel nauseated." But even if you don't have to report to a boss at the office or a grump-prone spouse at home, lots of walking is recommended as a stress reliever.

Many experts recommend walking for morning sickness and throughout pregnancy—especially if you've previously been sedentary. "Start at ten minutes, but if your legs hurt, skip a day," says Dr. Galloway. "Work up to 45 minutes a day, five days a week." Light weight lifting also helps stress, but be careful to *not* hold your breath while pumping iron.

WHAT CAUSES
MORNING SICKNESS?

Why does morning sickness afflict so many pregnant women?

Doctors know that it's caused by a hormone called estrogen that is rushed into peak production during your eighth or ninth week of pregnancy. It may be hard to believe while you're camped at the toilet, but morning sickness is actually a good sign. Studies show that women with morning sickness are less likely to miscarry or deliver prematurely. But even though it may be a good sign for your pregnancy, the nausea certainly doesn't feel good to you.

Relieve the pressure with acupressure. While a daily all-over body massage might sound ideal, Wataru Ohashi, founder of the Ohashi Institute in New York City, recommends this quick technique that he claims will cure or reduce morning sickness.

Ask for your partner's help with this. Either sit or lie down on your side, with your partner behind you. He should press his thumb down your back, first following the groove between your left shoulder blade and your spine, then keeping up the thumb pressure around the perimeter of your shoulder blade, moving out toward your side. Keep the pressure on for five to seven seconds at intervals along this path.

The pressure should be comfortable. If you feel a sore spot, ask your partner to keep his thumb there, giving that spot extra attention. Do the massage three times. Repeat the procedure down the right side. "If you stimulate the external, you can eliminate the internal discomfort," says Ohashi, who believes the trigger points you use in this exercise affect the stomach and the hormonal system.

Lift an hourly glass. Getting extra liquids is important if you've been vomiting, so drink several ounces of clear broth, water, fruit juice or flat ginger ale or cola every hour or so. When you feel queasy, a cup of raspberry leaf, chamomile or lemon balm herbal tea can help soothe your stomach.

"At the drugstore you can buy a high-carbohydrate nonprescription drink that helps: It's called Emetrol. It helps calm the emetic center, the portion of your brain that controls nausea," says Dr. Galloway. And sports drinks like Gatorade are also recommended, because they replace electrolytes—substances that regulate the body's electrochemical balance—that are lost when you vomit.

Trust your body's wisdom. "Eat whatever appeals to you, as long as you're not eating junk," says Gowen. "If all you crave is pasta, then eat it. It really does work when women listen to their bodies." The exceptions include sweets and other foods with "empty" calories, which can upset your stomach and trigger nausea. And doctors strongly recommend that you avoid caffeine, artificial sweeteners and fried foods.

Experiment. What worked for your sister, your best friend and the woman down the street may not do it for you. "There are as many remedies as there are women," says Deborah Gowen, a certified nurse-midwife with Women-Care in Cambridge, Massachusetts. You may have to try a couple of strategies before you find one right for you.

OSTEOPOROSIS

As you age, your bones erode a bit. That's normal. But some people lose so much bone that their skeletons become riddled with weak spots. That's osteoporosis, and it causes a lot of hip, spine and forearm fractures. At its worst, bones become so frail that they crack under the body's own weight!

Anyone can get osteoporosis, but women are more likely to get it than men. They have lighter bones than men, and they lose bone rapidly after menopause, because their bodies are producing less estrogen. But men aren't immune, especially if they drink heavily, smoke or have taken steroid drugs.

But your bones don't have to crack under the strain of this disease. You can slow, stop or even reverse bone loss. For women, medical treatment with estrogen replacement therapy (ERT) is the most effective way to accomplish this. But even if you choose ERT, there are natural methods to help it along. (And not surprisingly, they're the same tips and techniques that can help prevent osteoporosis in the first place.)

If you want to step lively and stall bone loss, here are the tactics doctors recommend.

Build those bones. "We suggest, as a minimum, that people follow the American College of Sports Medicine recommendations to exercise aerobically for 20 minutes a day at least three days a week," says Miriam Nelson, Ph.D., an exercise physiologist and research scientist at the U.S. Department of Agriculture (USDA) Human Nutrition Research Center on Aging at Tufts University in Boston. Exercise actually stimulates bones to lay down new tissue, she explains.

What's the best aerobic exercise for strong bones? "It's one you will continue doing, because if you don't do it *for life,* the bone-building benefits fade," Dr. Nelson says. In her studies, walking won top ratings—20 minutes a day three or four times a week—but you may prefer running, biking, swimming or aerobic dance classes.

Walk in water. If you've already had a fracture or two, your best choice of exercise may be walking in chest-deep water, working up to a half-hour at least three times a week, suggests Sydney Lou Bonnick, M.D., director of Osteoporosis Services at the Cooper Clinic in Dallas. The water will help support your body weight and take stress off bones and joints.

Make your "exercise equipment" a chair and the floor. To complement water walking, do some easy muscle-strengthening exercises in a chair or on the floor, suggests Mehrsheed Sinaki, M.D., a physiatrist in the Department of Physical Medicine and Rehabilitation at the Mayo Clinic in Rochester, Minnesota. Such exercises can include abdominal curls, shoulder blade squeezes and back extensions.

To do back extensions, lie on the floor on your stomach, with a pillow under your hips and your arms at your sides. Using only your back muscles, not your arms, raise your upper body a few inches off the floor. Hold for as long as comfortable, then relax downward. Work up to doing this six to ten times a day.

Chow down on calcium. Doctors agree that you should try to get 1,000 milligrams a day of calcium, even if you haven't reached menopause. And they suggest 1,200 to 1,500 milligrams a day for postmenopausal women who are not getting ERT.

Most women consume far less than those amounts. Reaching 1,000 milligrams through diet alone means drinking a quart of skim milk a day or eating two cups of low-fat yogurt or four cups of low-fat cottage cheese.

"Figure out, realistically, how much calcium you can get through your diet, then make up the rest with supplements," suggests Bess Dawson-Hughes, M.D., chief of the Calcium and Bone Metabolism Laboratory at the USDA Human Nutrition Research Center on Aging at Tufts.

Aim for maximum absorption. Spread your calcium supplements out over the day rather than taking them all at once, and take each one with a meal, Dr. Dawson-Hughes suggests.

Most doctors recommend calcium carbonate, a relatively inexpensive source of calcium that's fairly well absorbed if taken in divided dosages and with meals.

Get enough vitamin D. For maximum protection, aim for 400 international units (twice the Recommended Dietary Allowance), especially if you don't get much sun, suggests Dr. Dawson-Hughes. "Here in Boston, we tell people they need a more reliable source of vitamin D than the sun, especially during the winter months."

A cup of milk contains about 100 international units of vitamin D. But don't count on other dairy products, such as cheese, yogurt or ice cream, to fulfill your vitamin D needs. Unlike milk, these foods are not fortified with vitamin D.

Do not exceed the recommended dosage of 400 international units, however. Vitamin D is toxic in high amounts.

Graze far and wide. Bones are not made from calcium alone. They're an amalgam that includes zinc, boron and copper, among other minerals. "These trace elements are best gotten through a varied and broad-based diet that includes mostly unprocessed foods, such as whole grains, beans, fresh fruits and vegetables, fish and shellfish and lean meats," Dr. Dawson-Hughes says.

If you smoke, stop. "Smoking accelerates bone loss," Dr. Dawson-Hughes says. It speeds the rate at which the body metabolizes estrogen, virtually canceling out the bone-beneficial effects of estrogen replacement therapy. "And smoking must have other bone-rattling effects, too, because it causes bone loss in postmenopausal women not taking estrogen and in men," she adds.

Pass on the pop. Colas and some other carbonated soft drinks get their sharp taste from phosphoric acid, which contains phosphorus, a mineral that in excess amounts causes your body to excrete calcium.

STOP TRAINING FOR THE OLYMPICS

An intense exercise training schedule that leaves a woman so lean that she stops having menstrual periods also robs her bones of necessary calcium. "This usually happens only with elite female athletes, but it can also happen with women who are obsessed with staying thin and who exercise several hours a day," says Christine Wells, Ph.D., professor of exercise science at Arizona State University in Tempe.

The solution: "Aim for quality, not quantity, when you exercise. Train hard, eat well and maintain a weight that normalizes your menstrual periods," Dr. Wells recommends.

Salt lightly. As with phosphorus, too much salt causes your body to excrete calcium. So go easy on the shaker, and check food labels. Avoid products with more than 300 milligrams of salt per serving.

Monitor your medications. Some drugs can hasten bone loss, says B. Lawrence Riggs, M.D., president of the National Osteoporosis Foundation and professor of medical research at the Mayo Clinic in Rochester, Minnesota.

Those most likely to cause problems: corticosteroids, which are prescribed for a variety of conditions such as rheumatic disorders, allergic conditions and respiratory disease; L-thyroxine, a thyroid medication; and furosemide, a diuretic often used against fluid retention associated with high blood pressure and kidney problems.

"Talk with your doctor about this possible side effect," Dr. Riggs suggests. "If you have other risk factors as well, your doctor may want to check your bone density and, if it's low, alter the dosage or stop the drug entirely."

OVERWEIGHT

At this very moment, as many as one-half of *all* American adults are on a diet. Millions more are eagerly burning up calories with aerobics classes, clocking record mileage with walking or running or wearing out rowing machines and stair-climbers. All very serious enterprises when those extra pounds seem as though they're here to stay.

If you're among the more than one in three Americans who are overweight, you probably already know the keys to a slimmer body: a low-fat diet and regular exercise. But even with rice cakes and daily trips to the gym, those stubborn pounds may seem to stay around as long as deadbeat relatives on a long holiday. How come those pounds don't take a hint and *leave*?

Just wishing won't do the trick. But other methods will. Here's how you can speed up weight loss and make the most of your weight-control efforts.

Eat beans several times a week. "If you keep beans in your diet, you'll lose more weight, and you'll lose it faster," says Maria Simonson, Ph.D., Sc.D., professor emeritus and director of the Health, Weight and Stress Program at Johns Hopkins Medical Institutions in Baltimore. "That's because beans, which are very low in fat and calories, give you a feeling of fullness that can last up to *four hours longer* than meals without beans." Naturally, the more full you feel, the less likely you are to eat.

Drink more water. It's no secret that water is an effective weight-loss tool, and the more water you drink, the more weight you lose. Drinking a glass of water whenever you feel hungry helps take the edge off "food cravings," which often are actually cravings for fluid, says George Blackburn, M.D., Ph.D., chief of the Nutrition and Metabolism Laboratory at New England Deaconess Hospital in Boston. A glass before dining also helps you eat less.

Plan exercise around your meals. You probably know that aerobic exercise is essential to weight loss—even more impor-

THE SECRET OF SUCCESS: GET A NEW TABLECLOTH

P *ssst*, dieters, pay attention to the colors in your dining room: Choosing the right hues may help weight loss.

"Color influences the process of eating much more in the overweight than the underweight," says Maria Simonson, Ph.D., Sc.D., professor emeritus and director of the Health, Weight and Stress Program at the Johns Hopkins Medical Institutions in Baltimore, who *halved* her weight of 300-plus pounds before becoming a leading weight-loss researcher.

Her advice: "If you're overweight, get a tablecloth that's dark green, dark blue or coffee-colored brown, because it will help suppress your appetite." Painting your kitchen shades of dark blue, violet or green may also help.

And what has the opposite effect? Shades of orange, yellow and red tend to stimulate appetite and make us overeat—one reason why these are popular color choices in restaurants and most fast-food chains.

tant than diet, in fact, if you're over age 35. Still, many people don't know *when* to exercise to reap maximum benefits. The answer: light exercise after you eat.

Why? "A moderate workout after you eat uses just-consumed calories instead of storing them," says Bryant Stamford, Ph.D., director of the Health Promotion Center and professor of allied health at the University of Louisville School of Medicine in Kentucky. He points out that when you avoid storing calories, you also avoid turning them into fat. Dr. Stamford recommends an easy walk or other mild exercise *after* eating. You burn calories while digesting food, of course—but you'll *double* the calories burned if you get some exercise after the meal.

Lift weights to lower your weight. Although weight lifting has long been maligned as a second-rate fat burner (*aerobic* exercise takes the prize), new research indicates that the more muscle you have, the higher your metabolism rate. In fact, extra muscle makes your metabolism go up even when you're at rest.

Over the course of an 8- to 12-week weight-training program, you typically gain about three pounds of muscle. That extra muscle makes you burn an additional 250 calories a day, even when you're just sitting still, says Wayne Wescott, Ph.D., national strength-training consultant for the YMCA.

Make breakfast your biggest meal. Breakfast should *always* be your biggest and most caloric meal of the day. "You burn calories faster and more completely one hour after you wake up than at any other time of the day," says Dr. Simonson. She suggests that the single best dieting strategy is to eat a big meal before 9:00 A.M. every day, even if you aren't accustomed to eating a sizable breakfast.

Don't eat too *little*. Although many commercial diets call for 1,000 calories a day or less, experts say normal-weight women need at least 1,200 calories for long-term dieting success, and normal-weight men need about 1,500. Those calories are critical for good health.

"Ultra-low-calorie diets very rarely work over the long term," says Wayne Callaway, M.D., associate clinical professor at George Washington University Medical Center in Washington, D.C., and a member of the U.S. Dietary Guidelines Advisory Committee. "From a biological point of view, people on ultra-low-calorie diets are 'starving.'" When your body is that deprived, he says, your metabolism slows down—so you're really undermining the success of your weight-loss plan. It's also very difficult for your body to get all the nutrients it needs.

Dine to Dvořák. Listening to classical or other "soft" music during meals results in more chews per minute, according to studies at Johns Hopkins Medical Institutions. "People who eat fast often get hungry again soon after eating," says Dr. Simonson. If you take longer to complete a meal, you'll feel fuller and stay

FAT AND THE FUTURE

Obesity researchers have been no more successful than their patients in finding a cure for weight gain. It doesn't seem as though the future holds any hope for any techno-toner or cyber-slimmer that will melt off the pounds.

The required breakthrough must be a behavioral one, according to G. Kenneth Goodrick, Ph.D., an assistant professor in the Department of Medicine at Baylor College of Medicine in Houston. People have to overcome bad habits about inactivity and indulgent eating.

"We're set up as a society where it's easy to get high-fat food and difficult to exercise."

The food industry should play a continuing role by offering more nonfat alternatives, he suggests, and government can help by offering safe walking and jogging paths in parks.

feeling full for a longer time. "It's also easier to digest your food when you take longer to eat," she notes.

But stick to soft music: Hard-driving heavy metal and rock and roll can actually make you eat *faster*!

Seek out other pleasures. "A lot of people who think they want food really want pleasure, solace, comfort and relief from boredom," says Howard Flaks, M.D., an obesity specialist in Beverly Hills and chairman of public relations for the American Society of Bariatric Physicians. "Food is only one of an infinite number of pleasures."

Dr. Flaks gives his clients a list of 150 pleasures to try instead, such as taking a hot bath, calling a friend, getting a pedicure or planning a fantasy vacation. His advice: Instead of reaching for food, give yourself another pleasure.

PANIC ATTACKS

An upset stomach or chest pain could be this afternoon's lunch acting up. A racing heartbeat or shortness of breath could indicate you've exercised too much. Feeling "tingly" all over could suggest you're lucky at love.

The fact is, any of these symptoms could mean any number of things. But put them together—along with an almost uncontrollable feeling of impending doom—and it usually spells panic attack. Panic attacks are the primary symptom of panic disorder, which is one of the most common and more terrifying of all psychological disorders. These intense, unpredictable feelings of overwhelming anxiety and fear are so common that they affect an estimated 1 in 20 people.

Panic attacks vary in intensity and frequency, but they usually last from 5 minutes to an hour—averaging about 20 minutes. The typical sufferer gets them two to four times a week, but some people can get several in one day. "There are a lot of theories about what causes panic attacks: Some say it's genetic, others say it stems from childhood insecurity," says Christopher McCullough, Ph.D., a psychotherapist in Raleigh, North Carolina, and former director of the San Francisco Anxiety and Phobia Recovery Center. "But when you're having an attack, forget about insight and take care of the symptoms." Here's how.

Take a whiff of your childhood. Your nose knows—which is exactly why researchers urge you to sniff aromas that remind you of happy childhood memories. A sniff or two can almost *instantly* help curb fears and induce a more relaxed state—the first step in stopping a panic attack. "One odor that seems to work for just about everybody is baby powder," says Alan R. Hirsch, M.D., a psychiatrist and neurologist who heads the Smell and Taste Treatment and Research Foundation in Chicago. "Other odors have similar impact, depending on where you were born. Research shows us that for people from the East Coast, it's the smell of flowers. For those from the South, it's fresh air; in the Midwest, farm animals; and in the West, the smell of barbecuing meat." Other anxiety-easing smells include salt air, fresh-baked chocolate chip cookies and Mom's home cooking.

Stay active. "Probably the *worst* thing you can do is what most people tell you to do when you're in a state of panic—sit down and relax," says Dr. McCullough. "No matter what theory you have about the cause of panic attacks, at the point of the actual *attack*, it's a physiological event. It's all related to the sudden release of adrenaline—the fight-or-flight syndrome. So what you need to do is burn that adrenaline by exercising—taking a walk or moving around in some way."

Note: Studies show that people who practice a daily exercise program—rather than just when anxiety hits—bounce back faster in anxious situations.

Slow down your breathing. During a panic attack, you often hyperventilate—and that short and shallow gasping only adds to your state of fear. "You have to make a conscious effort to take long, deep diaphragmatic breaths," says Dr. McCullough. To practice deep diaphragmatic breathing, try to keep your chest and shoulders in position while you slowly expand and contract your stomach area.

Count backward from 100. "The purpose is to focus on *something* specific such as counting or touching, but not on your anxiety," says Jerilyn Ross, director of the Ross Center for Anxiety and Related Disorders in Washington, D.C., and president of the Anxiety Disorders Association of America. "Counting backward, counting the stripes on the wall, snapping a rubber band—doing anything that takes your mind off your panic attack helps, because it refocuses your thinking. You pay attention to things around you, rather than trying to fight the anxiety."

Get a massage. Particularly on the back of your neck, around your throat and in your diaphragm area, advises Dr. Mc-Cullough. "Those are the three areas where you can tense up because of anxiety. Rubbing your neck helps relieve tension, which

PHOBIAS: WHEN ANXIETY GOES AWRY

L et anxiety go out of control and it can result in a panic attack. Let the fear of having a panic attack get out of hand and you're likely to develop a phobia.

"A phobia is an involuntary fear reaction that usually revolves around a particular place or situation and is so intense that a person will do almost anything to get out of it," says Jerilyn Ross, director of the Ross Center for Anxiety and Related Disorders in Washington, D.C., and president of the Anxiety Disorders Association of America. "The important thing to understand about phobias is that the anticipating anxiety is usually worse than actually being in the 'scary' place or situation. The way to treat phobias is to gradually approach the situation you're afraid of and stay there long enough that the frightening feeling will pass. At the same time, refocus your thinking to positive thoughts. Each time you do this, you reinforce the fact that although the feelings are frightening, they are not dangerous. And that gives you courage to face the situation the next time."

can soothe or possibly prevent a panic attack, while breathing deeply relaxes the diaphragm area." When massaging the neck, massage only one side at a time. (If you rub both sides too enthusiastically, there's a risk you may cut off your blood supply and become unconscious.)

Remember that it's just a passing phase. No matter how scary a panic attack is, it helps to remember that it's only a passing phase. "You need to remind yourself that what you're feeling are normal bodily functions that are happening at the wrong time, and they're not going to hurt you," says Ross. "You're not going to die from it. You're not going crazy. And it will be over soon."

Don't leave your situation. It's not advised to run to get *away* from your fears, says Fred Wright, Ed.D., director of education for the University of Pennsylvania Hospital's Center for Cognitive Therapy in Philadelphia. "Escaping" your environment during a panic attack encourages the development of phobia—an irrational fear reaction to the place or situation you were in when the panic attack hit. Many of the people who have panic attacks eventually develop phobias, such as fear of driving, because they associate the attacks with a particular object or situation, rather than trying to remedy the anxiety itself.

Switch to decaf. People who get panic attacks are often highly sensitive to caffeine, says Alexander Bystritsky, M.D., assistant clinical professor of psychiatry and director of the Anxiety Disorders Program at the University of California, Los Angeles. So if you're prone to panic attacks, try to limit your intake of coffee, tea, chocolate and colas that contain caffeine.

Seek out support. You might want to consider joining a support group. If you can't find one, start one. The point of such groups is empowerment, says Meg McGarrah, former director of the Anxiety Disorders' Self-Help Group Network and author of *Help Yourself: A Guide to Organizing a Phobia Self-Help Group.* "It can provide companionship and information. Knowledge is power. A group helps you take charge of your recovery," she says.

PELVIC INFLAMMATORY DISEASE

Each year, thousands of women discover that they can't get pregnant—all because their fallopian tubes have been blocked by an often silent infection called pelvic inflammatory disease (PID).

The cause? Almost always it's a sexually transmitted disease, and often that disease is chlamydia, says Lisa Hirsch, M.D., assistant professor of obstetrics and gynecology and director of outpatient OBGYN services at the University of California, Irvine, Medical Center. Strictly speaking, when the same germs that cause sexually transmitted diseases in the vagina work their way up the cervix into the fallopian tubes, that's PID. Often, however, infections (even nonsexually transmitted ones) in the uterus, ovaries and cervix are also called PID. But you can lower your risk of contracting PID. In fact, this is one disease that is almost entirely preventable.

Preventing PID is relatively simple, but both you and your doctor have to be conscientious and aware, says Beverly A. Sansone, M.D., assistant clinical professor of obstetrics and gynecology at the University of California, Irvine, Medical Center and medical director of Planned Parenthood of Orange and San Bernadino counties. Dr. Sansone suggests how to avoid PID.

Practice safe sex. Preventing PID starts with preventing sexually transmitted diseases. That begins with smart sex. Yes, yes, using a condom can be tedious until you learn to include it as an integral part of sex. But it can help prevent sexually transmitted diseases, so it's a small price to pay to retain your fertility, says Dr. Sansone. The safest sex, of course, is to be had in a mutually monogamous relationship. Women who have multiple sexual partners have more than 4½ times the risk of getting PID compared with those in monogamous relationships.

Avoid intercourse if infected with a sexually transmitted disease. You don't want to spread a sexually transmitted disease to a loved one—nor do you want to give yourself PID. Intercourse can spread infectious germs upward to where they can cause PID. "We think that sometimes the bacteria hitch rides on the backs of sperm, which are carried up into the fallopian tubes," says Dr. Sansone. There's more to lovemaking than intercourse, and you don't need to refrain from affection.

Get checked immediately. The earlier PID is discovered and treated, the greater your chances of limiting harmful effects. "Doctors have to have a high index of suspicion to be able to detect PID," says Dr. Sansone. Although they're getting better, overall, "they still have to get more interested," she says. If you have reason to suspect PID and your doctor doesn't seem too concerned, find another doctor—a gynecologist is probably your best bet.

Make sure your partner gets checked, too. You and your partner, even if monogamous now, could have picked up infections before you began your relationship and could be passing them back and forth between the two of you. It makes no sense for you to get treated for PID if your partner is going to reinfect you. He should get checked for infection and be treated if necessary.

Take painkillers. Ibuprofen (Advil, Motrin), aspirin or acetaminophen (Tylenol) can relieve the pain and tenderness of PID.

Avoid sex. It may be too painful anyway, and you don't want to risk continuing reinfection from germs that haven't yet been killed by antibiotics or that come from an untreated sex partner.

Rest, eat well, drink plenty of fluids. "Treat yourself as if you had the flu," Dr. Sansone says. "Rest, fluids and food help your immune system help the antibiotics work. Much of the outcome depends on your own immunity."

PREGNANCY AFTER 35

According to the National Center for Health Statistics, the number of first births to women between 30 and 39 has more than doubled during the last 15 years. During the same period, there has been a 50 percent increase in the number of women over 40 giving birth for the first time. Ten years ago, a woman's biological clock began chiming when she was 30. Today, it may first strike when she is in her midthirties or even early forties.

What's extended the baby deadline? For one thing, it's become safer to wait. Prenatal testing has made it possible for a woman of 40 to reduce her risk of bearing a child with a genetic abnormality to that of a woman in her twenties. Technology has also spawned a vast array of treatments for infertility, which tends to increase in women over 35. And the new field of maternal/fetal medicine has allowed women with chronic illnesses and those who develop health problems during their pregnancies to deliver normal, healthy babies and survive pregnancy themselves. Relatively safe forms of contraception and public role models such as Bette Midler and Glenn Close—both first-time mothers in their forties—have also contributed to this pervasive it's-never-too-late attitude.

The truth is that many women have not deliberately delayed childbearing. Midlife pregnancy may simply be the side effect of infertility, marrying later or marrying for a second time.

PRIME-TIME CHILDBEARING

Although, medically speaking, the best time for a woman to have a baby is between the ages of 20 and 24, many feel that is not their emotional "prime time." For some women (and men) who grew up in the 1950s and 1960s, their twenties were more part of a prolonged adolescence than the anteroom of adulthood. In terms of childbearing, this shifting of adulthood has meant that women are peaking emotionally a decade, sometimes longer, after they peak physically. But the fact is, the "elderly primigravida" ain't what she used to be. Even the term, used in the medical textbooks, is becoming passé. Today a woman of 35 who becomes pregnant is not automatically "high risk." That's one less anxiety to face.

In fact, if a woman over 35 is physically healthy and has not had a history of infertility, miscarriage or stillbirth, her chances of having a normal, healthy baby are not significantly different from that of a 20-year-old, according to a study of 3,917 women who had babies at Mount Sinai Hospital in New York City. The study, headed by Gertrud S. Berkowitz, Ph.D., contradicted previous studies that found older women were more likely to have premature or smaller babies and babies who were more likely to die or have health problems.

Having a clear understanding of the real risks you face as an older, first-time mother is the first step to reducing stress during pregnancy, which can lead to labor and delivery complications, says Christiane Northrup, M.D., a gynecologist at Women to Women in Yarmouth, Maine, and co-president of the American Holistic Medical Association. "The worst thing for you, if you are healthy, is to be called high-risk, because the language alone may affect you psychologically. Every emotion is accompanied by changes in the body's biochemistry. If you think of yourself as sick, you can make yourself sick."

RETHINKING THE RISKS

A number of studies have suggested that what one doctor calls the obstetrical "nerve" factor may be at least partly responsible for the significantly higher cesarean rate for women over 35. In some cases, C-section rates are three times higher for older women than for younger women.

"Generations of obstetricians have been taught that maternal age is a risk factor," explains obstetrician and gynecologist Sally Faith Dorfman, M.D., commissioner of health in Orange County, New York. "If a woman is in her forties and having her first child, at the first sign of any problem the obstetrician isn't just going to sit there. She's going to want to intervene. Unfortunately, the studies of older pregnant women have been pretty biased and skewed. Years ago, older women who were delivering generally had one of two situations: Either they had already had many kids so their bodies might have been worn out, or they had tried for the last 15 years to conceive and had had a series of miscarriages."

More recent research, such as the Mount Sinai study, has focused on the more demographically current older mother who is likely to be middle class and well-educated, having a first, not a tenth, baby. When fertility factors are removed from the picture, the older woman and her younger sister aren't all that different.

And new obstetricians are being trained and medical textbooks are being rewritten, notes Dr. Dorfman. "I don't have the same kinds of prejudices as many other doctors," she explains. "I was born when my parents were 43."

OLDER AND WISER

It's becoming abundantly clear that older motherhood has some distinct advantages. In fact, when Wellesley College researchers Pamela Daniels and Kathy Weingarten asked a group of parents who had had children in their twenties if they would make the same decision again, more than half said that, given a second chance, they would wait. When the same question was posed to a group of parents who had waited until their thirties or forties to start a family, almost all said they thought their timing had been just right.

Women who wait are, truly, as ready as they'll ever be to take on the challenging task of bearing and raising children. Research has shown that older mothers are less likely to be ambivalent and have fewer conflicts about their pregnancies. In fact, they're likely to regard pregnancy as a blessing, and not simply because they've beaten the fertility odds. With age and experience comes knowledge—of who you are and what you want.

Pregnancy at midlife is usually the culmination of years of thoughtful consideration, the decision of two people of maturity and experience. Depending on the couple's age, it may be looked upon as a "last chance" and, therefore, as a precious gift.

"Research has shown that a child born to an older mother has a very special meaning for the mother, and older women are often less stressed and more open to and appreciative of the experience than younger mothers," says Ellen McGrath, Ph.D., executive director of the Psychology Center in Laguna Beach, California, who had the first of her two children when she was 40, the second at 43. "The child of the older mother comes into the world highly valued by a woman who is very clear on her values."

In a study done at Toronto General Hospital, comparing the feelings of older and younger first-time mothers, researchers found that the older women experienced less distress during their pregnancies than the younger women, despite the greater danger of having a child with genetic abnormalities and the perhaps more significant change a baby would mean in their lives. The researchers speculated that the older women, most of whom had married later in life, had, by virtue of their years, more opportunities to increase their feelings of self-esteem, confidence and independence, which contributed to their sense of well-being during pregnancy. Even though the women grew more depressed as labor approached, they were still less distressed than the younger women.

Also, the older woman, who has spent most of her adult life building her career, may see the pregnancy as a way to explore what is, for her, uncharted territory: Her femininity. "I see a lot of women, particularly women in their thirties who have had successful careers, who want to affirm the parts of themselves that have been dormant, that weren't brought out by simply being a wife or being in business," says Dr. McGrath. "For these women, having a baby represents the epitome of femininity. They feel they've had to keep the masculine sides of themselves dominant for so long in order to survive, they hunger for that kind of balance."

Unlike a younger woman who, perhaps, has still not made her mark on the world, the older mother is less likely to look to her child to fulfill her. She is also less likely to feel "held back" by a child while she tries to go about her unfinished business. Most older first-time mothers, have already taken care of business. "I remember my mother saying there were certain things she wanted to achieve in her life to prove she was as good as any man in her field, and she did, so she never had any resentment of children holding her back," says Dr. Dorfman.

GRAY-HAIRED MAMAS

Older parenthood has its downside, of course. Older mothers may not "bounce back" from childbirth as quickly as younger women. Some older women may also find it difficult to adjust to a demanding infant after decades of only looking after their own wants and needs. The woman who is highly organized may be caught short when everything from pregnancy to childbirth to mothering doesn't go according to plan, as often happens.

There are some other sobering realities to midlife pregnancy. Although it has been stretched, there is a childbearing deadline. Older parents may be forced to limit their families to one, or to space their children more closely than they may want to. Some critics of older parenthood have pointed out there is often a tendency among late-in-life parents to indulge their children—the too-precious child syndrome—particularly if the child is an "only." But that is by no means a tendency restricted to any one age group.

And there's some arithmetic to consider. At 35 or 40, a woman may find herself in a dual role: new mother and caretaker of her own aged parents.

And what kind of role models will gray-haired parents make to teenagers? Because of the wide age gap between parent and child, the potential for a virtual generation chasm is there.

In fact, while a younger mother may joke that "kids make you old," late-in-life mothers may find parenthood rejuvenating. Dr. Dorfman doesn't recall thinking of her mother as old. In fact, she says, she suspects many older parents find they're too busy to feel old.

"I remember asking my mother about menopause," says Dr. Dorfman. "She said, 'Hardly noticed it. I was too busy chasing 'young' thoughts and challenges from a 9-year-old, getting her to ballet lessons and Girl Scouts.' Late parenthood keeps you young. It keeps you vibrant and tuned-in. I saw it myself. When my parents' contemporaries were talking about retirement and moving to Florida, my mother was still active in the PTA!"

PREMENSTRUAL SYNDROME

Sugar and spice and *everything* nice? What about breast pain, bloating, weight gain and acne? Or cramping, headaches, food cravings and mood swings? When it comes to describing that aspect of womanhood known as premenstrual syndrome (PMS), nice isn't exactly the first word that pops to mind.

Common might be the word that better describes this complex of problems brought on by fluctuating hormone levels. About half of all American women between the ages of 20 and 50 have PMS, and upward of nine in ten women may experience at least some of its symptoms. But even though PMS brings on many kinds of discomfort, luckily there are also plenty of treatments.

Finding the best ones for you, however, may take some experimenting. PMS seems to be affected by stress, doctors say, and they agree that diet may be a large factor. So if the up-and-down symptoms of PMS are all too familiar, you might begin by looking at what's on your menu.

Get the saturated fat off your plate. Eating a lot of fatty foods will increase PMS symptoms and pain, according to Guy Abraham, M.D., a PMS researcher in Torrance, California, and former professor of obstetrics and gynecologic endocrinology at the University of California, Los Angeles. It helps to avoid fatty cuts of beef, lamb and pork. Better yet, substitute poultry and fish. And replace butter (which is high in saturated fat) with polyunsaturated oils such as flaxseed, corn and safflower, suggests Dr. Abraham.

Go without salt. "People don't realize that foods with a high salt content can contribute to water retention," says Susan Lark, M.D., medical director of the PMS and Menopause Self-Help Center in Los Altos, California.

Most snack foods and other processed foods are high in salt—

and some fast-food meals can be extremely high. So stay away from these foods if you're going on a low-salt diet, suggests Dr. Lark. Also, some boxed cereals and many condiments are higher in salt than many people realize. So read labels on packaged and processed foods, and whenever possible, choose fresh fruits and vegetables.

Counter the cravings with carbohydrates. Food cravings are common during PMS, and often those cravings focus on sweets and snacks such as ice cream, chocolate and potato chips. But you'll do yourself a favor if you can switch to other kinds of fare when you get the cravings.

"Eating complex carbohydrates such as whole grains, pasta, cereal and bagels is probably the best way to ward off food cravings experienced during PMS," says Dr. Lark. These foods also are a good source of fiber, which helps clear excess estrogen from your body, according to Dr. Lark. (High levels of the hormone estrogen have been shown to contribute to PMS.)

Eating high-carbohydrate, low-sugar foods provides another benefit as well, according to Judith Wurtman, Ph.D., a researcher at the Massachusetts Institute of Technology in Cambridge. She has found that cereal and other high-carbohydrate foods actually relieve the psychological symptoms of tension, anxiety and mood swings that accompany PMS.

Dr. Wurtman suggests having a heaping bowl of unsweetened cereal when you get hungry. (Reminder: Read the package label first, and choose a low-salt variety.) "It works like Valium," says Dr. Wurtman. In general, she has found, women who have PMS are more alert and happier when they eat high-carbohydrate foods rather than high-protein, low-carbohydrate foods.

Go for locomotion. When your mood takes a walk on the wild side, take a walk. "Exercising has been found to significantly reduce many physical and psychological PMS symptoms," says Ellen Yankauskas, M.D., director of the Women's Center for Family Health in Atascadero, California. That's because exercise releases endorphins, brain chemicals that ease pain and produce a sense of well-being. And in PMS sufferers, that means less crying and anxiety. Exercise has also been shown to help reduce breast tenderness, food cravings, fluid retention and depression.

"It's best to exercise at least three times a week, even when you don't have PMS," she says. "Walking is the exercise I recommend, because weight-bearing exercises help keep bones strong." She suggests going out for at least 12 minutes, though 30 minutes or more is even better.

Screen out foods with caffeine. If you happen to be caffeine-sensitive (and some people are more so than others), then you should avoid coffee, tea, colas and chocolate, according to Annette MacKay Rossignol, Sc.D., professor and chairman of the Department of Public Health at Oregon State University in Corvallis. Studies have suggested that the risk of PMS is between two and seven times greater in women who consume two or more cups of coffee or tea each day, according to Dr. Rossignol. Caffeine is a stimulant and can contribute to anxiety and irritability. Caffeine may also contribute to painful breast tenderness.

Read labels on pain relievers. Since caffeine can worsen PMS symptoms, you should make sure any pain relievers you take are caffeine-free. "You have to be a label reader," says Dr. Yankauskas. An over-the-counter pain reliever that contains caffeine can actually make your PMS symptoms worse.

Stay on the wagon. Alcohol is a depressant and diuretic that can worsen PMS headaches and fatigue and can accentuate depression, adds Dr. Yankauskas. For this reason, it's advisable to avoid drinking any alcoholic beverages, including wine or beer, when you've been having trouble with PMS, according to Dr. Yankauskas.

PROLAPSED UTERUS

"A prolapse is caused by a weakening of the supporting muscles and ligaments around the uterus, which makes it sag or slip down into the vagina, sometimes even reaching the vaginal opening," says Yvonne S. Thornton, M.D., associate professor of obstetrics and gynecology at Cornell University Medical College in New York City. "In some cases, bladder or bowel function can be affected, too.

"Having children through vaginal delivery is the most common cause of a prolapsed uterus," Dr. Thornton explains. "But the strain of simply carrying a child in the womb can cause it, too. Obesity and the chronic coughing common to cigarette smokers can also contribute to the problem."

How bad can it get? A prolapsed uterus can develop slowly over the years or appear suddenly. "It's different with different women," says Dr. Thornton. "You can go from no symptoms to seeing your cervix through your vagina in a rather short period of time. At that point it's called a third-degree prolapse, and it's very uncomfortable. Sexual intercourse becomes difficult because the penis is constantly bumping up against the cervix."

On the other hand, you may be unaware of your prolapsed uterus even during intercourse or when inserting a tampon. Some women have lived with the condition for 30 years or more before requiring attention for their symptoms. It just depends on how much discomfort you care to live with, says Dr. Thornton.

Embarrassing moments. Some women endure the discomfort until the last possible moment because it's so difficult to go to the doctor to complain about "this 'thing' between their legs," says Dr. Thornton. She says a woman is more inclined to come forward if her doctor is a woman. "At first, women are reluctant to talk about it because they find it embarrassing," she says. "Of course, I reassure them. After all, they're not responsible for their prolapse," she points out.

Depending on the severity of the prolapse, some women can't

even walk freely or do any of the sports activities that they did be-fore the prolapse. And sex can be a real problem. One woman ad-mitted to Dr. Thornton that she has to push her uterus back up with her finger before she and her husband can make love. No wonder it causes a lot of emotional stress.

What you can do. About 16 percent of all hysterectomies (and 33 percent for women over age 55) are done for uterine pro-lapse. But unless you have a third-degree prolapse, there are other less drastic options to consider—Kegels being tops on the list.

"Kegel exercises help strengthen your pelvic floor muscles, but you must do about 200 of them a day to notice an improvement if you have a prolapse," stresses Dr. Thornton.

Other options. Another nonsurgical option is a pessary—a ring-shaped device that fits around the cervix and props up the uterus. It's even effective for third-degree prolapses, says Dr. Thornton. But they are not without drawbacks. The pessary most commonly used today needs to be initially inserted by a doctor. It's deflated when you put it in, and then you inflate it to the point of comfort. They must be cleaned frequently and removed for intercourse. But if you're not sexually active or a good candi-date for surgery, this could be right for you.

There's also a surgical alternative that's not a hysterectomy. It involves resuspending the uterus in the abdomen. This is major surgery usually requiring general anesthesia, but if you want to save your uterus for any reason, you may want to consider it.

STRETCH MARKS

Since life is a series of trade-offs, it stands to reason that with every joyous event comes some downside: Experience the miracle of childbirth and you're bound to pay for it in some way—other than Junior's college tuition.

Stretch marks are as much a part of motherhood as Hallmark greeting cards, but even so, you don't necessarily have to carry them for the rest of your life. These cosmetic curses (particularly

---

WHEN RETIN-A WORKS, WHEN IT DOESN'T

Retin-A, which is available only with a doctor's prescription, has been getting a lot of attention for downplaying those nasty stretch marks. But there's a catch.

"The best time to use it is when the stretch marks are new—when they are pink and a little painful," says Melvin L. Elson, M.D., medical director of The Dermatology Center in Nashville, Tennessee, and the researcher who made the Retin-A/stretch mark connection. "If you wait until the marks become white, the success rate plummets from 80 percent to around 10 percent."

That means the prescription drug *must* be used within 6 to 12 weeks *after* getting the stretch marks—no later than three months after having a baby or losing a lot of weight. And Retin-A *cannot* be used during pregnancy or while you're breast-feeding.

As it does when used for wrinkles, the drug produces some initial skin irritation, peeling and redness at the application site. It works because it causes the "generation" of collagen, that all-important protein substance in the skin. Retin-A essentially performs a repair job, but you need to wait until the peeling and redness go away before you'll see its benefits. If a doctor does prescribe Retin-A, be sure to follow instructions carefully.

annoying come bikini season) are just harmless reminders that the human body isn't made of Play-Doh. And while pregnancy takes most of the blame for stretch marks, anyone can get them. Puberty, obesity and even weight loss are all common causes. Any time the body goes through drastic-enough physical changes, a skin protein substance called collagen can pull apart from the skin's elastic fibers, and that's when the telltale marks appear.

"They're basically nothing more than scars," says Stephen M. Purcell, D.O., chairman of the Department of Dermatology at Philadelphia College of Osteopathic Medicine and an assistant clinical professor at Hahnemann University School of Health Sciences in Philadelphia. So—what can you do about them?

If you go the doctor's prescription route, there's retinoin, a topical derivative of vitamin A marketed as Retin-A and best known for its effectiveness at erasing wrinkles. But for some people, home remedies *without* prescription might also get results.

Butter them up. "Although there's no scientific proof backing it up, some of my patients claim that rubbing on cocoa butter helps reduce or eliminate stretch marks—particularly in dark-skinned people," says Dr. Purcell.

Try hands-on healing. "We do know that massaging scars after surgery is beneficial, since it stimulates blood flow and distributes collagen more evenly, resulting in a less noticeable scar. So maybe that could work for stretch marks—and be the explanation behind cocoa butter," says Dr. Purcell. Maybe it's the massaging action, not cocoa butter, that gets rid of stretch marks.

TOXIC SHOCK SYNDROME

I n 1980, the federal Centers for Disease Control (CDC) in Atlanta began receiving reports of a mysterious, sometimes deadly disease striking hundreds of women. The women, investigators soon learned, had several things in common. Most were between the ages of 18 and 52. Most were having their periods when they became ill. And most were using high-absorbency tampons.

Experts called the disease toxic shock syndrome. While not a new disease, investigators eventually linked the sudden outbreak of cases to the use of high-absorbency tampons and especially to one particular brand of super-absorbent tampon. In fact, when these super-absorbent tampons were removed from the market, the incidence of toxic shock syndrome declined as quickly as it had appeared. But it has not disappeared.

What is this dangerous disease, and what does it have to do with tampons?

A SHOCK TO THE SYSTEM

Toxic shock syndrome occurs when a strain of staphylococcus bacteria—or, more precisely, poisons produced by staph—gets inside the body. It may follow skin infections, childbirth or surgical procedures, but in a majority of cases, it gets in through the vagina—usually during menstruation when tampons are used.

In the early stages, toxic shock syndrome may cause fever, vomiting, diarrhea and muscle aches, says Ken Zangwill, M.D., a medical epidemiologist at the CDC. Without medical attention, however, toxic shock syndrome can be, quite literally, toxic. Approximately 6 percent of these cases are fatal, says Dr. Zangwill.

The bacteria that cause toxic shock are common. "Staph may be found on the skin, in the nose and throat and in other mucous membranes," says Dr. Zangwill. It's not entirely clear why staph infections, which usually are mild, will on occasion produce toxic shock syndrome.

The link with menstruation isn't entirely clear either, Dr. Zangwill says. It's possible that tampons, by drying the inside of the vagina, create a favorable environment for staph. It has also been suggested that inserting and removing tampons may very slightly damage the vaginal lining. "This could potentially allow the organism to penetrate and get into the body," says Dr. Zangwill.

REDUCING THE RISKS

Though toxic shock syndrome can be extremely serious, the risks of actually getting it are extremely low, says Dr. Zangwill. "Toxic shock is a rare disease, even among tampon users."

To lower the risks still further:

Abandon tampons. Since toxic shock syndrome usually occurs in tampon users, switching to sanitary napkins—which don't irritate the vagina—will help prevent it. Even using tampons less often can help, says Dr. Zangwill. For example, some women use tampons during the day, then switch to sanitary napkins at night.

Avoid "super" tampons. According to the CDC, each 1-gram increase in tampon absorbency increases the risk for toxic shock by 37 percent. In other words, a "super" tampon that absorbs 9 grams of fluid can be *111 percent* more risky than a "slender," which absorbs no more than 6 grams. Doctors recommend women use the least absorbent tampon that still is adequate for their needs.

The Food and Drug Administration requires tampon manufacturers to list absorbency ranges on the outside of packages. If you're not sure which tampons are right for you, ask your doctor or pharmacist for help.

ACTION ALERT

If you do suspect toxic shock, fast action can be a lifesaver. That's why it's so important to watch out for symptoms. If while menstruating you have a high fever (more than 102°F) and are

TOXIC SHOCK SYNDROME— IT'S NOT FOR WOMEN ONLY

Toxic shock syndrome has come to be associated with women and menstrual periods to the extent that some call it "the tampon disease."

But women aren't the only ones who can get toxic shock syndrome. Researchers say toxic shock can befall anyone infected with the bacterium *Staphylococcus aurens*. While this type of bacterial infection may strike menstruating women, it may also occur in surgical incisions or burns. Early symptoms to watch for include a rash, fever, diarrhea and vomiting.

vomiting and having diarrhea, remove the tampon and see your doctor *immediately*.

Toxic shock syndrome always requires hospitalization, Dr. Zangwill says. Since the disease usually is accompanied by severe fluid losses through vomiting and diarrhea, most people will require fluid replacement therapy. They'll also get antibiotics.

When leaving the hospital, most people take with them a 10- to 14-day supply of antibiotics. After two weeks, the infection— and the danger—should be gone.

URINARY INCONTINENCE

It's a problem many people are reluctant to mention, even to their doctors. And that's unfortunate, because *nearly everyone* who temporarily loses control of their bladder can be made better or cured, experts agree.

"Most people who have incontinence can be helped, and that includes the elderly," says Catherine DuBeau, M.D., an instructor in medicine at Harvard Medical School and a member of the Gerontology Division and the Continence Center at Brigham and Women's Hospital, all in Boston.

First of all, Dr. DuBeau points out, "it's important to have a medical evaluation to determine what kind of incontinence you have and what's causing it." During the evaluation, your doctor will suggest which treatments might work best for you. While drugs or surgery are sometimes called for, there are many other approaches that doctors recommend. Here are some of them.

Get on a schedule. Follow the clock as you schedule times to go to the toilet. Most people start by going every hour or so for a few days; then, if they remain dry, they go on a two-hour schedule. If you feel an urge to go in between times, stop and relax, then walk slowly to the toilet. The goal is to go every three or four hours during waking hours, Dr. DuBeau says. "What you're doing, in a sense, is trying to retrain the brain to control the bladder, so it doesn't contract unless you are on the toilet, ready to go." People on this daytime program are less likely to get the sudden urge to go at night, she observes, because the bladder is trained for a regular schedule.

Learn the Kegel squeeze. These exercises strengthen the pelvic floor muscles, which contract and relax to control the opening and closing of your bladder. When they are weak, urine may leak out when you sneeze, laugh, contract your abdomen, lift something heavy or simply get up out of a chair, explains Katherine

F. Jeter, Ed.D., executive director of Help for Incontinent People (HIP) in Union, South Carolina, and assistant clinical professor of urology at the Medical University of South Carolina in Charleston.

This kind of wetting problem, called *stress* incontinence, often improves with Kegel exercises, Dr. Jeter says. "Doing these exercises regularly can build up pelvic muscle strength and, in some cases, help you regain bladder control."

First identify the muscles you'll be exercising: Without tensing the muscles of your legs, buttocks or abdomen, imagine you are trying to hold back a bowel movement by tightening the ring of muscles around the anus. Do this exercise only until you identify the back part of the pelvic muscles.

Next, when you're passing urine, try to stop the flow, then restart it. This will help you identify the front part of the pelvic floor.

Now you're ready for the complete exercise. Working from back to front, pull up and tighten the muscles while counting to four slowly, then release and relax and count to four slowly. Do this for two minutes at least three times daily, for a total of approximately 40 to 50 repetitions.

If you're doing Kegel exercises right, expect improvement in a few weeks to months, Dr. Jeter says. If you're not certain you're doing them correctly, talk to your doctor or nurse.

For people who have stress incontinence, it helps to do a Kegel squeeze before you cough, laugh, get out of a chair or pick up something heavy. The muscle contractions help prevent wetting accidents.

Drop some weight. "Obesity does seem to make bladder control more difficult, and we've had letters from people who say they've lost weight and improved bladder control," says Cheryle B. Gartley, president of the Simon Foundation for Continence in Evanston, Illinois, and editor of the book *Managing Incontinence*.

Retire your pogo stick. Bouncy exercises don't cause stress incontinence, but in people who already have a problem, they can cause leakage, Gartley says. Learning Kegel exercises can help solve the problem for many. Don't avoid exercise, she advises, but try the kinds that are less jarring. Gartley often recommends swimming or biking.

Stay regular. If you're constipated, take steps to get your bowels moving. Constipation can impair bladder control, Dr. DuBeau says.

When you go, make sure you empty your bladder completely. Remain on the toilet until you feel your bladder is empty. If you feel there is still some urine in the bladder, stand up, sit back down, and lean foward slightly over your knees.

Check the drugs you're taking. "There are a host of medications that can contribute to urinary incontinence," says Dr. DuBeau. "We ask people to make a list of all the medications they take, including over-the-counter drugs. One of the first things we do is review that list. Antihistamines, antidepressants, even common pain relievers such as ibuprofen [Advil] can cause problems. It's extremely important to let your doctor know about any medication you are taking."

Keep a food diary. Coffee, milk, sugar, corn syrup, honey, alcoholic beverages, tea, soft drinks, chocolate, citrus juices and fruits, tomatoes or tomato-based products and highly spiced foods have all been associated with incontinence in some people, Dr. Jeter says. To find out whether incontinence follows consumption of certain foods, try going without one kind of food or drink for a week or so. If that helps, it's a sign that you should continue to keep that food off your diet.

URINARY TRACT INFECTIONS

They danced in Greek *tavernas*, raced from the bulls in Pamplona and nibbled goat cheese in Corsica. Altogether a perfect honeymoon—until the new Mrs. Drabble started going to the bathroom 15 times a day. She went twice during breakfast, three times during lunch and six times during supper—and that was before her evening espresso! "My dear, let us talk of love," crooned the dashing Mr. Drabble, thinking only of romance as the full moon rose and reflected in the sparkling sea. "Excuse me," sighed Mrs. Drabble, eyeing the ladies room. "I'll be right back!"

MARAUDING MICROBES

Urinary tract infections (UTIs) often come at the worst times, says Joshua Hoffman, M.D., an internist in private practice in Sacramento, California. It's very common for infection-causing bacteria in and around the vagina to be "massaged" into the urethra, the tube that extends to the bladder, during intercourse. That's why doctors sometimes refer to UTIs as "honeymoon cystitis."

More than 80 percent of all UTIs are caused by bacteria that originate in the intestine and live quite comfortably and, most of the time, harmlessly in the area near the anus. Trouble begins when they migrate—during sex, for example—into the urethra. In women, the anus and the urethra are close together, so it's relatively easy for bacteria to make the trip. Men, with their extra inches of anatomy, rarely are affected. That's why UTIs often are considered a woman's problem.

Of course, you don't have to be on your honeymoon, or even be sexually active, to experience the aching, burning and frequent urination that commonly accompany a UTI. At least one out of three women will eventually contract a UTI, and women who are particularly susceptible get three, four, even five a year, Dr. Hoffman says.

UTIs can occur anywhere in your urinary tract. An infection in your bladder is called cystitis; in your urethra, urethritis; in your kidneys, pyelonephritis. While pyelonephritis can be quite serious, most UTIs are easily treated, Dr. Hoffman says. Even if you do nothing, your body's natural defenses will usually clear things up. Call your doctor if your condition doesn't improve within 24 to 48 hours, says Dr. Hoffman.

BEATING THE BUGS

If you've had one UTI, you'd prefer never to have another. Women with recurrent UTIs can stop the vicious cycle with preventive maintenance, says Dr. Hoffman. Here's how.

Flush them out. It's entirely normal to wake up in the morning with bacteria in your bladder, Dr. Hoffman says. You don't even know they're there. But if you start the day without urinating, those few invaders have time to multiply rapidly. A few hundred can turn into thousands in no time. Flushing them out will prevent them from gathering enough forces for a successful attack. But a good defense means more than emptying your bladder when you wake up. You have to keep the flow going all day long.

"There are a few bugs in your urinary tract almost all the time, but when you urinate, you wash them out," Dr. Hoffman explains. To keep your bladder—and urethra and kidneys—bacteria-free, you have to keep fluids moving. The more water you drink, the more you urinate. The more you urinate, the lower your chances for picking up an infection.

You should drink at least six to eight glasses of water a day. Water and fruit juices are preferred over most other liquids such as soft drinks, which can contain salt that inhibits urination.

Caution: If you're already taking antibiotics for a UTI, too much water can make them less effective. Ask your doctor how much water you should drink during and after your therapy.

Infectious interruptus. Because bacteria always are in and around the vagina, it's difficult to prevent them from getting

ANTIBIOTICS TO THE RESCUE

Antibiotics are so effective at curing a urinary tract infection (UTI) that some doctors are prescribing them as a preventive for women plagued with recurrent attacks. According to researchers at the University of Washington School of Medicine in Seattle, daily antibiotics can be highly effective in preventing UTIs, even when taken for as long as five years. And they don't appear to cause antibiotic-resistant strains of bacteria, which often is a risk with the long-term use of antibiotics.

Another study done by researchers at the same school found that while some women may benefit from taking antibiotics every day, others can take them only as needed—after intercourse, for example, when they're more at risk for contracting an infection. In the study, researchers looked at two groups of women prone to UTIs. One group took antibiotics after they had intercourse. The other took placebos (blank pills). Of the 16 women who took postcoital antibiotics, only two (12.5 percent) developed a UTI. Of the 11 women taking placebos, nine (81.8 percent) developed infections.

Doctors typically are cautious about the long-term use of antibiotics. For one thing, bacteria adapt to their environment. They can also change very quickly—sometimes in days or even hours. When bacteria are exposed to antibiotics in less-than-lethal doses, they can develop particularly virulent strains that are hard to kill. What's more, antibiotics can sometimes cause unpleasant, even dangerous, side effects.

But the bacteria that cause UTIs usually are fairly predictable and easy to get rid of. Used in low doses both to treat UTIs and to prevent them, antibiotics are quite safe, says Sacramento, California, internist Joshua Hoffman, M.D. "Antibiotics are concentrated in the urine, which is why urinary tract infections are easy to prevent," Dr. Hoffman says. "You can use small doses of antibiotics, which turn out to be a very large concentration in the bladder, and that knocks the bacteria out."

into the urethra during intercourse. But you can flush them out by going to the bathroom after sex, Dr. Hoffman suggests.

Wipe away. Left to themselves, the bacteria in the periurethral area—that is, in the area near the urethra—like to stay at home. But if you push them toward the urethra, you're courting a UTI. "After a bowel movement, wipe the rectal area toward the *back* and the urethral area separately toward the *front*," Dr. Hoffman says.

Be a bad host. If your urine is sweet and nice, it'll attract bacteria. If you make it acidy and inhospitable, bacteria will hit the road. "High doses of vitamin C can help acidify urine," Dr. Hoffman says. "In combination with lots of fluids, that may help prevent some UTIs."

If you have problems with recurrent UTIs, you might want to ask your doctor about vitamin C therapy. Although vitamin C is not toxic, high dosage of any vitamin should only be taken under the supervision of a doctor. Long-term use of high doses of vitamin C can cause digestive problems such as diarrhea. You can get plenty of extra vitamin C naturally by increasing your intake of citrus fruits and certain green vegetables such as broccoli and kale.

The cranberry connection. Some doctors believe there may be some merit to this folk remedy, although no one has come up with a universally acceptable answer as to why it may work. One theory suggests that cranberry juice may contain chemicals that prevent infection-causing bacteria from clinging to the urinary tract. Some say it simply helps boost vitamin C intake. At the very least, it will boost your fluid intake and help flush bacteria from your system, Dr. Hoffman says.

Diaphragm dangers. Some women who use a diaphragm are particularly prone to UTIs, perhaps because it gives bacteria two more chances—during insertion and removal—to get inside. If you get frequent infections, ask your doctor if another type of birth control might be more appropriate for you.

VAGINAL DRYNESS

I t's hard to determine which aches more because of this condition—your vagina or your feelings. Sex becomes a lot less fun if you lack the natural lubrication to enjoy lovemaking. In fact, it may get downright painful. But there's also the self-doubt, depression and even anger that you and your partner might feel because of it.

Instead of blaming yourself (or him), you might want to point the finger at a lack of estrogen. During menopause, you can *expect* estrogen to be in short supply. But if that's not the only reason for the problem, other causes might include a low-grade vaginal infection, taking birth control pills or even the natural aging process. Besides getting estrogen replacement therapy from your doctor, here are some natural ways to make intercourse go more smoothly.

Toss out the cigs. "Smoking destroys estrogen in the body," says Ellen Yankauskas, M.D., director of the Women's Center for Family Health in Atascadero, California. Since the most common cause of vaginal dryness is lack of enough estrogen, smoking only makes the problem worse.

Choose the right lubricant. You can remedy vaginal dryness with a commercial lubricant, but avoid anything scented or oil-based. "You want a lubricant that's water-soluble, unscented, colorless, odorless and tasteless," says John Willems, M.D., associate clinical professor of obstetrics and gynecology at the University of California, San Diego, and a researcher at the Scripps Clinic and Research Foundation in La Jolla. "After that, it's a matter of personal choice." He and other experts recommend Astroglide, SurgiLube, Lubrin vaginal inserts, Gyne Moisturin and the more familiar K-Y jelly. Another recommended product is Replens, a moisturizer that can be used on a regular basis.

The key is to stay away from oil-based products like petroleum jelly or cocoa butter—or homemade recipes. "Some people use whatever is on the night table—things like suntan oil," says

Dr. Willems. "But they aren't good for the vagina and can cause problems."

Go for fatty acids. Eating foods that are rich in fatty acids can be a big help. Among the best sources are raw pumpkin, sesame and sunflower seeds. Also eat fish that contain lots of fatty acids: Salmon, tuna and mackerel are all good choices, because they help retain estrogen in the body, says Susan Lark, M.D., medical director of the PMS and Menopause Self-Help Center in Los Altos, California.

Don't douche. Most douche products have a drying effect, which contributes to vaginal dryness, adds Dr. Yankauskas. "In general, you shouldn't douche unless you feel it's absolutely necessary—and it's usually not."

Savor the moment. "Give yourself more time for foreplay," suggests Dr. Willems. As women age, he points out, their response to sexual stimulus is slower. You don't lose sexual response—it just occurs at a different pace.

Get professional help. "If vaginal dryness leads to bleeding or intense itching, these signs should be looked at by your gynecologist," says Yvonne Thornton, M.D., professor of clinical obstetrics and gynecology at Columbia University College of Physicians and Surgeons in New York City. They could be an indication of more serious problems.

VAGINITIS

As most women can attest, any itching or discomfort in the vaginal area is just one nuisance too many. Unfortunately, this area is a regular magnet for trouble. The dark, moist surroundings are the perfect breeding ground for a wide array of bacteria and other organisms that can cause a host of irritations, inflammations and infections.

"Vaginitis is basically a catch-all phrase for any kind of inflammation of the vaginal area," says Ellen Yankauskas, M.D., director of the Women's Center for Family Health in Atascadero, California. "Inflammations can result from an infection, a chemical irritation from douche products, spermicides or condoms or simply not having enough estrogen." Whatever the cause—and there are many—here are some cures.

Obey the Zen Commandments. Women with recurring vaginitis might want to consider a usually unlikely suspect—stress. "For chronic cases, I ask the woman to breathe deeply and try to get completely relaxed, so she can ask herself what she needs to know," says Susan Doughty, R.N., who is a nurse practitioner at Women to Women, a clinic in Yarmouth, Maine.

In Doughty's view, a regular, meditation-like evaluation of yourself can answer "internal" questions that could be subconsciously causing physical symptoms. Doughty also recommends looking at relationships: "We can keep treating the infections, but there's usually some issue in a woman's relationship with her sexual partner that needs to be addressed."

Practice brand loyalty in birth control. "Many women notice vaginitis when they switch brands of condoms or spermicides," says Dr. Yankauskas. "If you notice an irritation or infection after trying one brand, then obviously it's not the one for you." But, if you're not having any problems with a brand, stay with it.

Go thigh-high in stockings. Panty hose may be a fashion godsend, but they're a contributing cause of vaginitis and yeast in-

A SOLUTION FOR SOME MONTHLY PROBLEMS

Some women experience vaginal itching just prior to their menstrual flow. Once their period ends, the itching seems to stop until the following month, observes Susan Doughty, R.N., a nurse practitioner at Women to Women, a clinic in Yarmouth, Maine. Your doctor may tell you that this condition, cytolytic vaginosis, is caused by an overgrowth of bacteria in the presence of estrogen. Since this is just an imbalance (not a true infection), you may be able to clear it up with a home-prepared remedy.

The remedy, according to Doughty: Mix two tablespoons of baking soda in one quart of warm water and douche twice daily. The first douching should be just before the time of the month when symptoms typically appear. After that, continue to douche twice daily as long as you have the symptoms.

After a few months, reassess whether you need to continue, suggests Doughty. You don't need to use the douche again unless the itching returns.

fections. "Panty hose do not allow the skin to breathe," says Dr. Yankauskas. When the crotch area is covered by panty hose, it becomes a better breeding ground for infections. "If you must wear stockings, I recommend the thigh-high types rather than the full cover-your-crotch styles," says Dr. Yankauskas.

She and other experts also recommend wearing only cotton panties—and not blends—because cotton allows for better air circulation.

Double-rinse your underwear. Harsh laundry detergents can increase the amount of irritation that results from vaginitis, says John Willems, M.D., associate clinical professor of obstetrics and gynecology at the University of California, San Diego, and a researcher at the Scripps Clinic and Research Foundation in La Jolla. So make sure all detergents and soaps are thoroughly rinsed from underwear.

Favor *bambino's* soap. "If you're prone to vaginitis, or when you have an irritation, use the same soaps to bathe with as you would use on a baby," says Dr. Yankauskas. "Avoid deodorant soaps or anything with heavy dyes and perfumes."

***Don't* treat it with yogurt!** While the yogurt/yeast infection connection is known far and wide, realize that yeast infection is only *one* type of vaginitis—and yogurt may not be the cure. "Some women try to treat vaginitis with a tampon dipped in yogurt," says Doughty, "but if the infection is bacterial, it'll grow like crazy when it comes in contact with yogurt."

Be careful with chemistry. Certain chemicals can cause what appears to be a vaginal infection, says Dorothy Barbo, M.D., professor of obstetrics and gynecology at the University of New Mexico School of Medicine and medical director of the university's Center for Women's Health in Albuquerque. "Some women become allergic to douches or the perfumes or deodorants that they contain, she says. "Occasionally, I've seen women who have developed an allergy to tampons, to latex condoms or to the spermicide that's used with a diaphragm. Although the symptoms may feel like a yeast infection, there is no sign of the fungus upon examination. What you've got then is an inflammation of the vaginal area. Simply eliminating what's triggering the inflammation will often solve the problem."

VARICOSE VEINS

Many people deal with varicose or "spider" veins the same way: with a cover-up. When those reddish or blue bulges appear on legs and thighs, there's a temptation to buy a wardrobe full of long skirts and pants and pretend this isn't happening.

But guess what? Many of the people you're hiding your legs from also have varicose veins. No fewer than 10 percent of men and 20 percent of women have varicose veins or the less prominent, weblike, spider veins that show up on the thigh. That means more than 20 million Americans in all are involved in this cover-up.

Sometimes varicose and spider veins can be quite painful, but it's reassuring to know they usually are *not* serious and don't lead to other problems in the legs or circulatory system. You can't change the veins, but you *can* ease the pain. Here's what the experts recommend.

Take an aspirin every day. "One of the easiest ways to get relief is to take half an aspirin every morning and every night," says Luis Navarro, M.D., founder and director of the Vein Treatment Center and senior clinical instructor of surgery at Mount Sinai School of Medicine, both in New York City. "Not only does aspirin help relieve any pain you might have from varicose veins, it also increases blood mobility."

Tilt your bed. One simple remedy is to place bricks or blocks of wood under your bed's footboard, so your feet will be raised a few inches, suggests Andrew Lazar, M.D., assistant professor of clinical dermatology at Northwestern University Medical School in Chicago. But check with your doctor first if you have a history of heart trouble or difficulty breathing during the night.

Learn yoga. A simple yoga breathing practice can help relieve varicose vein pain, says John Clarke, M.D., a cardiologist with the Himalayan International Institute of Yoga Science and Philosophy in Honesdale, Pennsylvania. Simply lie flat on your back and prop your feet up on a chair. Breathe slowly by expanding your diaphragm—that is, the whole area just *under* your lungs. (With diaphragmatic breathing, your stomach should rise and fall.) While doing this, breathe through your nose. In this position, gravity pulls excess blood out of your raised legs, and your full, steady inhalations create negative pressure in your chest, Dr. Clarke says. This negative pressure helps pull air into the chest cavity, which also helps get the blood flowing from your legs into the trunk area of your body.

Put up your feet—a lot. Weakened veins lack the strength to return blood to the heart. Since veins in your legs are farthest from the heart, you're helping them out whenever you get gravity on your side.

For one exercise that brings relief, lie flat on your back, raise your legs straight up in the air, and rest them against a wall for two minutes. Or simply place your legs on an easy chair to raise them above hip level whenever they're aching. Using either of these leg-raising methods, the discomfort should start to go away, says Dudley Phillips, M.D., a family practitioner in Darlington, Maryland.

Get those legs moving. "Any exercise that helps strengthen the legs can help varicose veins," says Dr. Navarro. "That's because when muscles contract, their compression empties the superficial veins and sends the blood to the deep veins and toward the heart." Although some reports claim that bicycling and running *worsen* varicose veins, Dr. Navarro says that applies only to excessive amounts of exercise. "Unless you're a professional athlete, *any* exercise will help," he says.

Watch your salt intake. Salt in the diet contributes to swelling, says Dr. Navarro. "So if you have a propensity toward swelling, you're better off restricting the amount of salt you consume." Avoid salting your meals, and look for low-salt or sodium-free packaged products. And watch out for fast food that's usually high in salt.

And watch your weight. Added body weight, especially excess abdominal fat, creates more pressure on your groin; this makes it harder for venous blood to return to the heart. Keep your weight down and chances are you'll have fewer problems with bulging veins, says Lenise Banse, M.D., a dermatologist and director of the Northeast Family Dermatology Center near Detroit.

Avoid constriction. Girdles and other constricting clothing can act like tourniquets and keep blood pooled in your legs. If you have varicose veins, it's advisable to wear loose-fitting clothing and give up knee highs.

Stock up on special stockings. Support stockings and compression stockings, available in pharmacies and department stores, resist the blood's tendency to pool in the small blood vessels closest to the skin, says Dr. Phillips. When you wear these stockings, the blood is pushed into the larger, deeper veins, where it is more easily pumped back up to the heart. Compression stockings exert twice as much pressure as support stockings. Dr. Navarro suggests you choose a pair with a rating of 20 to 25 millimeters of mercury compression. The higher the compression, the greater the support these stockings provide. But there is a trade-off: Stockings with higher compression are less comfortable to wear.

WATER RETENTION

When you feel as though you're too big for your skin, not to mention your britches, check for some other signs. Perhaps your face is puffy, especially when you first wake up. Your ring may feel tight, and your belly seems bloated. Do your shoes feel like they belong to Minnie Mouse? Does this awful, bloated, uncomfortable feeling seem to come out of the blue? What is going on?

It could be water retention, or *edema* (to use the medical name). It happens to all of us to some extent during a normal 24-hour period, says Norman C. Staub, M.D., a professor in the Department of Physiology at the University of California, San Francisco. "Our bodies are constantly adjusting fluid levels based on what we drink and eat."

Usually our bodies do an admirable job of quickly correcting fluid balance. But sometimes the balance gets temporarily thrown off. Too much salt or alcohol, long periods of inactivity and, for women, monthly hormone fluctuations or pregnancy can all tip the scale toward fluid retention. A sudden weight gain of several pounds may be your first and only sign that you're retaining fluid. Swollen ankles are a common tip-off, too.

For mild fluid retention, here's what experts suggest.

Get into deep water. As any skin diver knows, water pressure forces fluid out of tissues and, ultimately, into the bladder. You can get similar results by exercising in a swimming pool, according to Vern L. Katz, M.D., associate professor of obstetrics and gynecology at the University of North Carolina Medical School at Chapel Hill. Try a half-hour, three times a week, of gentle water exercise in a pool that's 80° to 90°F, or about skin temperature. "Avoid water above 100° if you're pregnant," Dr. Katz warns.

Avoid using diuretics. While they're very effective at removing excess body fluid for patients who have heart, kidney or liver disease, diuretics set up the potential for something called rebound edema, says Robert Schrier, M.D., a professor and chairman of the Department of Medicine at the University of Colorado School of Medicine in Denver. If you're taking them steadily for minor fluid retention, the diuretics turn on a lot of salt- and water-retaining hormones, says Dr. Schrier. "When you stop taking them, the high levels of hormones cause a lot more sodium and water retention, and you get into a vicious cycle."

Shake the salt habit. Too much salt—from hot dogs, popcorn, olives, salted nuts, pickles or pepperoni pizza—makes your body retain fluid. That fluid stays with you until your kidneys have a chance to excrete the excess salt, which can take about 24 hours. So if you avoid salty foods, you are less likely to have noticeable fluid retention, Dr. Staub says.

While you're at it, shake a leg. Exercise can relieve the body of excess fluid and salt through sweating, increased respiration and, ultimately, increased urine flow, Dr. Staub says. Walking up and down the hallway, or climbing a flight of stairs every hour or so, will reduce the fluid retention you develop from sitting for long periods of time. If you must sit still, try this: Point your toes downward, then raise them up as high as you can. That pumps your calf and your foot muscles. Moving your arms around up over your head will help, too.

Drink plenty of water. Water moves through your kidneys and bladder, diluting the urine. And since urine has some fluid-retaining salt in it, the more it's diluted, the easier it is to remove salt and prevent or decrease edema.

"Plain water is definitely the best, because just about every other drink—juices, soda, milk— has salt in it," Dr. Staub says.

Sip an herbal tea. Several herbs have a mildly diuretic effect, according to William J. Keller, Ph.D., a professor and head of the Division of Medicinal Chemistry and Pharmaceutics at Northeast Louisiana University School of Pharmacy in Monroe. Parsley is the best known of these. Try two teaspoons of dried leaves per cup of boiling water. Steep for ten minutes. Drink up to three cups a day.

Lie down, put up your feet. Sometimes this is the simplest and best thing to do, Dr. Staub says. If you recline with your feet in a raised position, you allow fluid that has pooled in your legs to more easily make its way into the circulatory system and then to your kidneys, where it can be excreted.

Beware the warning signs. Occasionally fluid balance gets seriously thrown off. Heart and kidney problems, along with other serious diseases, can cause life-threatening fluid retention. Don't delay seeing your doctor if you have a sudden weight gain, swollen ankles or difficulty breathing.

If you find that an indentation remains when you press your skin, that's a sign of "pitting edema"—a type of fluid buildup that needs a doctor's attention.

WRINKLES

A lot of good can come with age—things like wisdom, grandchildren and senior citizen discounts. But there are a few not-so-terrific things, like gray hair and wrinkles.

Gray hair, of course, can be touched up with a little dye. Simple enough. Wrinkles, however, are an altogether different story. No, you can't iron them out. And you can't (like Peter Pan or Dorian Gray) simply wish them away. But experts say there are a number of strategies to keep you from looking old before your time.

Sleep on your back. "You can create wrinkles by sleeping on your side or belly, with your face on the pillow," says D'Anne Kleinsmith, M.D., a cosmetic dermatologist at William Beaumont Hospital near Detroit and a member of the American Academy of Dermatology who is an expert on wrinkles. "You'll see this in people who have a diagonal crease on their forehead, running above their eyebrows. For some people, sleeping on their back eliminates this problem."

Take your vitamins. The best vitamins for your skin are B-complex vitamins, found in beef, chicken, eggs and whole wheat, and antioxidants—vitamins A, C and E—which are abundant in green leafy vegetables, carrots and fresh fruit. These vitamins help ensure healthy and young-looking skin, says Marianne O'Donoghue, M.D., associate professor of dermatology at Rush–St. Luke's–Presbyterian Medical Center in Chicago.

Stop the squint with shades. "One problem area for wrinkles is around the eyes—what we call crow's feet," says Dr. Kleinsmith. "These wrinkles often result from squinting, so one way to avoid them, or lessen their severity, is to wear sunglasses when you go outside."

Keep a stone face. "Excessive frowning or smiling, or any other much-repeated facial expression, emphasizes wrinkles," adds

Dr. Kleinsmith. "I'm not saying you should not smile or frown, but try to be aware of how often you're doing it—especially frowning." She and other experts advise *against* facial exercises, because excessive facial contortions only "aggravate" wrinkles.

Don't open another pack. Smoking is a double whammy for wrinkles. "Smokers have more wrinkles than people who don't smoke, especially around their lips," says Dr. Kleinsmith. That's because smoking robs the complexion of oxygen, decreasing blood circulation to facial skin and resulting in premature lines and wrinkles. *Plus,* anyone puffing on a cigarette is essentially doing a lot of repetitive facial movements that add even more wrinkles.

Go light on the bottle. The sobering fact is, excessive drinking causes your face to "puff up" the morning after, which temporarily stretches the skin. Subsequent shrinking brings your face back to normal but also causes wrinkles, says Gerald Imber, M.D., a plastic surgeon at The New York Hospital–Cornell Medical Center in New York City.

Avoid the midday sun. It's no surprise that too much sun exposure is the leading cause of premature wrinkles. The trouble is, no one except Count Dracula can avoid the sun all the time. But take note: About 95 percent of the sun's wrinkling rays occur when Old Man Sol is at his strongest—between 10:00 A.M. and 3:00 P.M.—says Stephen Kurtin, M.D., assistant professor of dermatology at Mount Sinai School of Medicine in New York City. As long as you avoid those maximum-intensity hours, you're doing your skin a favor.

Ban the tanning booth. Whether it's achieved indoors or out, today's tan leads to tomorrow's wrinkles. The synthetic sunshine found in tanning booths is just as bad as the real thing, wrinkle-wise, says Jeffrey H. Binstock, M.D., assistant clinical professor of dermatologic surgery at the University of California, San Francisco, School of Medicine.

WHEN YOU SHOULD WEAR EGG ON YOUR FACE

Big night out? Just because you want to paint the town doesn't mean you have to get ready by painting your face with expensive wrinkle-hiding creams. Here's a way to avoid the cosmetic shelf and still have smoother-looking skin.

"It will only last a couple of hours, but a couple of egg whites work as well as those $100-an-ounce wrinkle creams," says Jerome Z. Litt, M.D., a dermatologist and assistant clinical professor of dermatology at Case Western Reserve University School of Medicine in Cleveland. "You beat the egg whites—not the yolks—into a meringue and put it all over your face just before your party. Leave it on for about 30 minutes and then wash it off with cool water. [*Don't* use hot water or you'll have scrambled egg all over your face!] Pat your face dry, and then go off to your party."

Dr. Litt says the protein in the egg whites helps tighten the skin. "There's nothing permanent about it, but it does help for an hour or two. It's also effective for shrinking pores," he says.

Wash with the cool and mild. Excessive washing and scrubbing—particularly with hot water and harsh soaps—tends to dissolve oils that help nourish the skin, says Jerome Z. Litt, M.D., a dermatologist and assistant clinical professor of dermatology at Case Western Reserve University School of Medicine in Cleveland. Dr. Litt says to wash with cool or lukewarm water, using a mild soap or cleanser such as Neutrogena soap or Moisturel sensitive skin cleanser.

Use a moisturizer. If you have dry skin, daily use of a moisturizing lotion can temporarily help hide smaller wrinkles that form on the skin surface, says Dr. Kurtin.

YEAST INFECTIONS

I t takes very little to get the normally docile *Candida albicans* fungus that lives in a woman's vagina to turn into a rampant troublemaker. Candida is encouraged by many things—getting pregnant, using spermicides or birth control pills or taking antibiotics. And if you nick the vaginal walls while inserting a tampon, that can also trigger this most common form of vaginitis.

Yeast infections are not dangerous, but they can be painful and embarrassing. The most common symptoms include a bothersome itch and burning that can become maddening. Often there's a white discharge that resembles cottage cheese, sometimes accompanied by a yeasty or fishy smell. Here's how to cease the yeast.

Watch your sweet tooth. Sugar can cause chronic yeast infections—which is one reason why women who binge on sweets are particularly prone. "Avoid candy, cakes and pies—anything with refined, white or powdered sugar," says Jack Galloway, M.D., clinical professor of obstetrics and gynecology at the University of Southern California School of Medicine in Los Angeles. If you must indulge your sweet tooth, use brown sugar or honey. Since these take longer to break down in your body, you'll lessen the amount of circulating blood sugars, which can trigger yeast infections.

And watch the rest of your diet. Take heed of the connection between yeast infections and yeasty foods. "Avoid things such as bread, mushrooms and alcoholic beverages," says Susan Doughty, R.N., a nurse practitioner at Women to Women, a clinic in Yarmouth, Maine. She says that patients with chronic yeast infections who avoid these foods for three to six months will often notice a significant improvement.

"C" an improvement. Eat plenty of foods that are high in vitamin C, such as potatoes, citrus fruits and broccoli, adds Dr.

Galloway. Vitamin C helps boost your immune system, and "if your immunity is down, you're a prime candidate for a yeast infection."

Wear baggy clothing. Tight-fitting clothing doesn't allow for good air circulation in the vaginal area. So stay away from clingy polyester, Lycra spandex, leather and other fabrics that don't "breathe." "Yeast love it when it's moist, dark and warm," says John Willems, M.D., associate clinical professor of obstetrics and gynecology at the University of California, San Diego, and a researcher at the Scripps Clinic and Research Foundation in La Jolla.

If you must wear tight clothing or Lycra, do it for only a few hours—and then change into loose-fitting garb made from cotton and other natural fibers. Dr. Willems says to avoid panty hose when you can, because they're too restrictive in the vaginal area.

Change wet clothing fast. Lounging around in a wet bathing suit? You're wearing a perfect environment for yeast growth, adds Dr. Galloway. So once you're out of the pool, change into a dry outfit.

Heal with yogurt. Most experts point to yogurt as *the* natural healer of yeast infections (though it shouldn't be used for other types of vaginitis). Yogurt's lactobacillus cultures fight the candida, says Eileen Hilton, M.D., an infectious disease specialist at Long Island Jewish Medical Center in New Hyde Park, New York, who has studied yogurt's effect on yeast infections. While some experts recommend inserting yogurt into the vaginal area, an easier way is to simply eat at least ½ cup of yogurt containing live cultures each day to prevent and treat infections. (Nearly all yogurt *does* contain live cultures.)

"If you don't like the taste of yogurt, you can get a dose of the same helpful bacteria by drinking milk containing live lactobacillus," says Ellen Yankauskas, M.D., director of the Women's Center for Family Health in Atascadero, California. (This type of milk will be identified on the container as cultured milk, acidophilus milk or kefir milk.)

TAKE YEAST INFECTIONS TO THE CLEANERS

Perhaps the best weapons for treating yeast infections are in your laundry room. But you have to use special tactics to conquer *Candida albicans*, which can survive regular wash-and-dry cycles. Here are the basics.

- Go soak. Soak panties in water for a half-hour or more before washing them.
- Scrub-a-dub-dub. After soaking, scrub the crotch of your panties with unscented detergent before putting them into the washing machine, advises candida specialist Marjorie Crandall, Ph.D., of Yeast Consulting Services in Torrance, California.
- Double-rinse. Make sure panties are rinsed thoroughly: residues from soaps and detergents can intensify vaginitis, adds John Willems, M.D., of the University of California, San Diego.
- Get 'em hot. Studies have found that the heat-sensitive candida die when panties are touched up with a hot iron.

Sit in a sitz. Frequent douching should be avoided, since it can be too irritating to those with yeast infections. But there's an easy cleansing solution for your vaginal area. Fill the bathtub to hip height with warm water, then add ½ cup of salt (enough to make the water taste salty) and ½ cup of vinegar. Stay in this sitz for about 20 minutes.

Go for a nonprescription medication. "The best way to treat this infection is with an over-the-counter antiyeast vaginal cream," according to Dr. Yankauskas. The creams are available in most pharmacies. Just follow the directions on the package.

Give applicators a hot scrub. If you use an antiyeast cream, you're probably reusing the applicator. "Wash the reusable applicators in hot soapy water," says Dr. Galloway.

Try no-frills toiletries. Avoid bubble baths, scented tampons, colored toilet paper and other products with dyes, perfumes and other chemicals that can irritate vaginal tissue, says Dr. Willems. White toilet paper is your best bet.

And don't dust. Starch is the perfect medium for growing fungus cultures, says Michael Spence, M.D., an obstetrician and gynecologist at Hahnemann University School of Medicine in Philadelphia. Since most after-bath powders have a starch base, you're encouraging an infection when you use a dusting powder.

Put spermicides in their place. Spermicides are another chemical to keep out of your vagina, especially if you are prone to infections. If you plan to use a spermicide during intercourse, put the spermicide inside the reservoir tip of the condom, where it can do the work it was meant to do, says Marjorie Crandall, Ph.D., a candida specialist and founder of Yeast Consulting Services in Torrance, California.

Choose natural fibers first. Use cotton tampons instead of synthetic fiber tampons. Superabsorbant tampons and those left in more than 12 hours will stop natural drainage and encourage bacterial growth. Another idea: Use pads at night and tampons during the day.

Sleep like Eve. Yeast thrives in a warm, damp atmosphere, says Dr. Spence, so one of the best preventive measures you can take against this fungus is to keep your vaginal area ventilated—that is, cool and dry. Sleep naked or take your panties off underneath your nightgown when you go to bed and give your body 8 hours of unencumbered relief.

INDEX

Note: <u>Underscored</u> page references indicate boxed text.